The Complete Vegan & Vegetarian Cookbook

2 Books in 1: Discover The Health Benefits of Eating a Plant Based Diet With 170 Easy, Quick and Flexible Recipes For Changing Your Nutrition Plan

Richard Tillcot

Table Of Contents

Vegan Curried Rice

Vegan-Friendly Falafel

Simple Vegan Icing

Penne with Vegan Arrabbiata Sauce

Kingman's Vegan Zucchini Bread

Vegan Red Lentil Soup

Vegan Lemon Poppy Scones

Bold Vegan Chili

Vegan Hot and Sour Soup

Vegan Banana Blueberry Muffins

Spicy Vegan Potato Curry

Vegan Brownies

World's Best Vegan Pancakes

Vegan Corn Bread

Quick Vegan Spaghetti Sauce

Vegan Corn Muffins

Vegan Potatoes au Gratin

Vegan Split Pea Soup II

Vegan-Friendly Caramel Buttercream

Vegan Bean Taco Filling

Vegan Split Pea Soup I

Vegan Agave Cornbread Muffins

Vegan Cupcakes

Spicy Thai Vegan Burger

Vegan Fajitas

Vegan Gelatin

Vegan Cheesecake

Vegan Borscht

Vegan Yogurt Sundae

Vegan Pumpkin Ice Cream

Vegan Chunky Chili

Vegan Lasagna II

Vegan Carrot Cake

Vegan Mexican Stew

Tangy Vegan Crockpot Corn Chowder

Traditional Style Vegan Shepherd's Pie

Yummy Vegan Pesto Classico

Vegan Baked Beans

Delicious Vegan Hot Chocolate

Vegan Cream 'Cheese' Frosting

Easy Vegan Pasta Sauce

Vegan Goddess Dressing

Vegan Mac and No Cheese

Vegan Pumpkin Nog

Vegan Chili

Vegan Sun-Dried Tomato Pesto

BOOK 2: VEGETARIAN DIET COOKBOOK 2021

Introduction

How to Become a Vegetarian

Vegetarian Weight Loss Diet

Being a Vegetarian

Vegetarian Sports Nutrition

Low Carb Vegetarian

Vegan Vegetarian

97 Best Vegetarian Recipes

Easy Vegetarian Red Beans Lasagna

Spicy Vegetarian Lasagna

Rae's Vegetarian Chili

Vegetarian Cabbage Rolls

Vegetarian Purple Potatoes with Onions and Mushrooms

Vegetarian Carrot Cake

Vegetarian Penne

Vegetarian Pasta

One Dish Vegetarian Dinner

Vegetarian Quiche

Italian Vegetarian Patties

Vegetarian Black Bean Chili

Vegetarian Bean Curry

Vegetarian Cake

Lucie's Vegetarian Chili

Vegetarian Lime Orzo

Vegetarian Sweet and Sour Meatballs

Vegetarian Meatloaf

Vegetarian Stuffed Peppers

Vegetarian's Delight Pizza

Vegetarian Meatloaf with Vegetables

Vegetarian Baked Pasta

Vegetarian Refried Beans

Vegetarian Tortilla Soup

Vegetarian Four Cheese Lasagna

Vegetarian Tortilla Stew

Vegetarian Moroccan Stew

Vegetarian Faux Chicken Patties

Easy Vegetarian Corn Chowder

Nut Burgers (Vegetarian)

Vegetarian Brown Rice Casserole

Hariton's 'Famous' Vegetarian Casserole

Vegetarian Shepherd's Pie II

Unbelievably Easy and Delicious Vegetarian Chili

Veggie Vegetarian Chili

Vegetarian Jambalaya

Southwestern Vegetarian Pasta

Vegetarian Stuffing

Insanely Easy Vegetarian Chili

Fire Roasted Vegetarian Gumbo

Vegetarian Lentil Spaghetti

Vegetarian Shepherd's Pie I

Vegetarian Mushroom-Walnut Meatloaf

Vegetarian Sandwich Spread

Vegetarian Cassoulet

Vegetarian Lasagna

Easy Vegetarian Pasta

Vegetarian Green Chile Stew

Vegetarian Gravy

Delightful Indian Coconut Vegetarian Curry in the Slow Cooker

Summer Vegetarian Chili

Vegetarian Tortilla Dog

Malaysian Quinoa (Vegetarian)

Vegetarian Chickpea Sandwich Filling

Vegetarian Sloppy Joe's

Vibrant Vegetarian Purple Borscht

Vegetarian Turkey Stuffing

Vegetarian Burrito Casserole

Grandma's Slow Cooker Vegetarian Chili

Vegetarian Nori Rolls

Clinton's Special Vegetarian Quiche

Vegetarian Haggis

Vegetarian Stuffed Red Bell Peppers

Vegetarian Kofta Kabobs

Vegetarian Split Pea Soup

Vegetarian Spaghetti

Vietnamese Style Vegetarian Curry Soup

Vegetarian Kale Soup

Vegetarian Ribs

Vegetarian Stuffed Poblano Peppers

Al's Quick Vegetarian Spaghetti

Vegetarian Chili

Sunday Vegetarian Strata

Easy Vegetarian Stroganoff

Vegetarian Tourtiere

Vegetarian Buffalo Chicken Dip

Vegetarian Pasties

Vegetarian Link Gravy

Vegetarian Chili

Vegetarian Open Faced Sandwich

Vegetarian Chickpea Curry with Turnips

Vegetarian Southwest One-Pot Dinner

Meatiest Vegetarian Chili from your Slow Cooker

Vegetarian Moussaka

Vegetarian Phad Thai

Vegetarian Pate

Vegetarian Shepherd's Pie

Vegetarian Nut Loaf

Alissa's Vegetarian Lentil Meatloaf

Vegetarian Korma

Vegetarian White Bean 'Alfredo' with Linguine

Vegetarian Cottage Cheese Patties

Convenient Vegetarian Lasagna

Vegetarian Reubens

Farmer's Market Vegetarian Quesadillas

Vegetarian Stuffing

The Best Vegetarian Chili in the World

The Complete Vegan Cookbook For Beginners

Discover The Health Benefits of Eating a Plant Based Diet: Over 70 Quick, Easy, Inspired and Flexible Recipes For Changing Your Nutrition Plan

Richard Tillcot

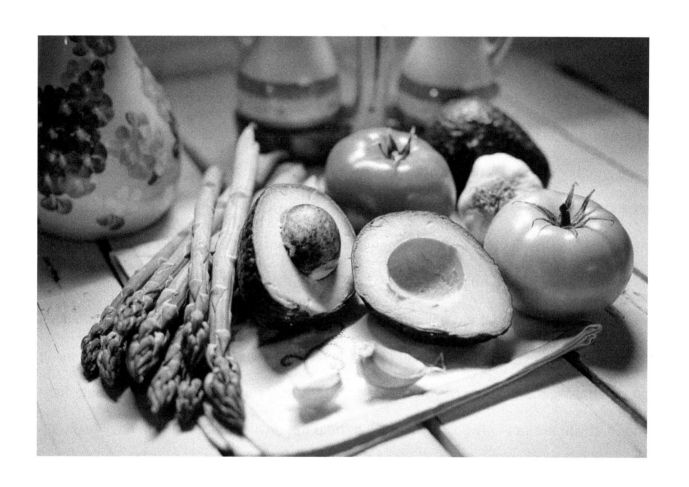

LET'S START!

Reasons to Embark in Vegan Cooking

With so many people around the world looking to embark on a greener lifestyle it is no wonder that the Vegan lifestyle is receiving a large amount of attention lately as well. From people who are looking to embark in just some minor changes to those who are looking to completely revamp their entire lifestyle. Regardless of whether you are looking to make a massive change or just a few small differences Vegan cooking can offer a large number of benefits, which helps to ensure that many people start picking up the habits.

Aside from the reality that a Vegan lifestyle is much more green friendly than eating tons of meat it also has a huge benefit of being a much cheaper lifestyle. Because the majority of the foods that are eaten in a Vegan lifestyle can be grown at home it provides a substantial savings that you would not otherwise be able to realize if you were relying on purchasing the majority of your foods from a grocery store. By omitting meats from your diet you are not only doing your part to help the environment but with savings in the thousands of dollars possible each year it can be a huge benefit to look towards a Vegan lifestyle.

Other concerns that are important is the ability to avoid chemical treated foods. Many Vegans opt to grow their own produce, which provides the huge benefit of allowing you to use your own home grown organic foods. This makes them much cheaper for you, which again can significantly decrease your average grocery bill.

It is still very important to realize that you might need to buy some food items from the store, however you will not need to worry about the items that you do need to purchase as much since the costs will be significantly lower and there are generally less likely to be subject to harmful chemicals.

Many people opt to turn to a Vegan lifestyle due to the health benefits. It is a proven reality that people who consume large amounts of meat tend to weigh more. This is a reality that cannot be avoided especially due to the increasingly large number of people around the world who are becoming obese. By changing to a Vegan lifestyle, it is much easier to lose weight and find a much healthier lifestyle that will benefit your entire family. In order to really see the benefits of this it is necessary that you take some time to really devote to the Vegan lifestyle to see a real benefit.

There are some studies lately that speculate that Vegan cooking has been linked to also help reduce the occurrence of diabetes as well. In order to really know if this is true for you it is important to talk to your doctor. Many people experience huge changes to their blood sugar levels by switching to a Vegan lifestyle, however many others also find that it is increasingly difficult to find a good method of changing their blood sugar levels to reduce the need for additional medication. If you are looking to reduce your blood sugar levels then it is important to talk to your doctor before making the adjustment.

With any change you might be considering you should always take plenty of time to review your options. Most people find that the Vegan lifestyle is perfect for their needs without spending months of research however; you should still take at least a bit of time to ensure that this is the right lifestyle for you. If you are not interested in making a permanent change then you should consider making some small changes and working to tweak each of these changes to your exact lifestyle preference. You might need to make several changes, but you should be able to settle into a comfortable pattern and lifestyle quite quickly if you devote a bit of time and effort to the process.

The very first step you need to take is a good accurate assessment of your current cooking skills. If the idea of walking into the kitchen to cook has you sweating profusely then you are again not alone, but it will mean that you need to come to terms with the kitchen. If your idea of cooking is running to the local take out and putting food on plates or even eating straight out of the box you will again need to come to terms with the kitchen. A vegan diet is possible, but while eating out is also possible it is not as healthy, nor will you find the same amount of options as you can prepare yourself at home.

Another first step that you should take is always look for the help and support of your family. If you are going to be embarking on a change such as switching to a Vegan lifestyle, you need the support of your family to help you out. If you have them on board to make the change with you it will be much easier for everyone to provide support and encouragement. However, it is also extremely important that you take some time to really review all of your options and ensure that recipes that you select will be enjoyable for everyone. Many people make the mistake of picking only recipes that they enjoy, which leaves the rest of their family left out.

To embark on a truly Vegan lifestyle is a very important decision that should never be taken lightly. Simply rushing into the experience can have devastating results. If you are careful and make a wise decision for your family, you will find that the benefits of Vegan cooking are wonderful. A few well planned cooking classes and a bit of additional effort placed into creating meals and it will be no time at all before you are completely satisfied with the delicious dishes that a Vegan lifestyle can provide for you. This makes it a great way to get into a healthier state and also encourage better eating habits.

Top Tips for Vegan Cooking

In the beginning, you might discover that Vegan cooking is more of a pain and hassle than it is a benefit. If you discover yourself in this position, you are not alone. However, there is help available for you. Taking some time to really look over all of your options is best to ensure that you are able to get the biggest benefit possible from the healthier lifestyle. Vegan cooking is something that will typically require you to think carefully as well as plan ahead, in this spirit it is extremely important to be sure that you are getting everything planned out ahead of time to ensure you have what you need.

One of the biggest suggestions to get the biggest benefit is to look into cooking with the fruits and vegetables that you like the most. If you have a serious objection to eating okra for example you should never dash out and look for a stack of okra recipes. Instead, you need to focus on the recipes that involve ingredients that you like. Of course, a bit of trying new foods is always good, but building a base of foods that you like is a great starting point.

To ensure that your new Vegan diet is as affordable as possible you need to look for fruits and vegetables that are in season to cook. If you are constantly having to purchase expensive fruits and vegetables for your meals you will quickly discover that your budget is blown far before it is time to even work on the next months budget. Spreading your money around as much as possible will demand that you buy only foods that are in season as much as possible.

If you are truly interested in living the ultimate Vegan lifestyle, it is time to start investing in a garden for your house. You do not need to dedicate acres of space to the garden, but a small area to raise at least the basic vegetables would be considered essential.

If you can spare some additional space to add some more vegetables then go right ahead, however never feel as if a garden is wasted if you only have a few feet. To start with you need to look towards tomatoes and even peppers. These are both extremely easy to grow, take very little space and can save a bundle of money. Having your own fresh vegetables to eat is a huge perk.

Look for ways to save as much money as possible. If you are going to embrace a Vegan lifestyle, you should reap all of the benefits. This means looking for some pick your own farms, which will allow you to pick your own produce at a significant savings. If you are only buying small batches of produce you will discover that it can quickly turn expensive. Purchasing larger supplies can provide you ample stock to enjoy fresh foods as well as allow you to can or freeze additional supplies to have for the off-season months.

A final suggestion to follow as you are getting started with Vegan cooking is to look for some great cooking classes designed to start teaching from the very basics. This will allow you to learn numerous ways to cook without the problem of your meals tasting plain and boring. If you are truly interested in exploring a delicious Vegan lifestyle then the cooking classes are something that you will have to venture into. An alternative to the classes would be to stop by a friend's house and get some cooking tips from them, this however is only effective if your friend is also a Vegan and can teach you some of the best tips and tricks for retaining flavor and producing delicious meals. Working to live a healthy lifestyle does not involve boring meals that you suffer through; rather with some practice you can create truly remarkable dishes.

7 super-foods for vegan athletes

Veganism is a concept that deals with abstaining from the consumption of animal-based products such as milk, eggs and meat. Vegans follow a strict vegetarian diet minus dairy products. Vegans are only allowed to consume vegetables, fruits, grains, legumes, nuts and seeds.

Now you might think that this does not sound like an ideal diet for athletes to follow, as most of them rely on animal protein like meats and eggs to develop a strong body. However, the world of veganism can offer several superfoods that are not only great to develop a strong body but also capable of increasing an athlete's vitality.

If you are a vegan athlete, then you have come to the right place, as we will look at 7 such superfoods that can be incorporated into your daily diet.

1) BERRIES

Kick-starting the list of vegan superfoods are berries! Berries happen to be one of the most recommended foods for athletes and for good reason. Berries can offer the body several benefits that are highlighted as shown below:

Muscle recovery

Berries are credited for increasing muscle recovery. This means that they help in reducing the time taken by your body to recover from muscle tears and soreness. According to an experiment conducted on athletes, where they were given blueberry smoothies before their workout, they were able to recover better from muscle soreness 60 hours after their session.

Oxidative stress

The same experiment also found that berries greatly reduced oxidative stress as blood samples drawn 60 hours post workout showed less cell damage. An athlete releases more free radicals into the body after a workout session. Berries, being rich in antioxidants, have the power of reversing oxidative damage to a large extent. This is quite important when it comes to maintaining not just muscle health but overall wellness.

Fat cell development

Berries help in inhibiting fat cell development. Fat cells need to be controlled in order to prevent fat deposits from accumulating in the body. As per studies conducted on mice, those that chewed on polyphenols- a nutrient present in berries- saw a 73% decrease in their lipids. This goes to show that berries can truly help in curbing fat deposits in the body.

Metabolic syndrome

Berries are said to help in the fight against metabolic syndrome. This syndrome can induce reduced metabolism, inflammation, glucose intolerance, insulin resistance etc. Those who are unable to exercise long hours will see a marked improvement in their stamina after consuming berries.

Here are some berries to add to your daily diet.

• Acai berry

Being rich in antioxidant properties, Acai berries are great for athletes.

Most athletes suffer from immense pain after a workout session owing to the buildup of lactic acid. Berries help in cutting down on this acid thereby reducing the pain.

• Blueberries

Blueberries are said to be the king of berries and are a must for all athletes to include in their diet. Blueberries come with extreme anti-oxidant content and a chemical known as Lactate dehydrogenase that helps in reducing oxidative damage. This, in turn, helps in enhancing muscle health and help athletes' recover faster from muscle tears and soreness.

• Goji berries

Goji berries help in increasing cellular respiration. This means that your cells will have more oxygen before and after a workout thereby enabling better performance. These berries also contain Lactate dehydrogenase, thereby making them a must have in your diet.

As you can see, nibbling on a few berries before and after your workout can help in increasing your athletic performance to a large extent.

2) OATMEAL

It is no secret that oatmeal is considered to be a favorite breakfast all over the world. It keeps you full and provides your body with lots of fiber. However, these are just minor benefits compared to the ones that they are capable of providing athletes.

Oatmeal is quite a popular ingredient in a body builder's diet and makes for an important component of daily meals. It need not always be consumed for breakfast and can be eaten as a pre/post workout snack. Here are some of the reasons that make oatmeal ideal for athletes.

B vitamins

One important vitamin that is essential for the upkeep of muscle health and metabolism are B vitamins. B vitamins include vitamin B6, B7, B3 and B5, all of which are required to improve muscle function. A single cup of oats is capable of providing your body with the requisite amount of B vitamins and increasing muscle recovery. You will also feel energetic for several hours without having to snack in between.

Magnesium

An important component of an athlete's diet is magnesium. Magnesium is required to relieve sore muscles, enhance cell repair and cut down on the stress hormone known as cortisol. Magnesium also helps in maintaining a healthy nervous system. A single cup of cooked oats can leave you with 275 milligrams of magnesium, much more than what several vegan foods combined can offer.

Proteins

It's a no-brainer that athletes require proteins to build stronger muscles. Proteins help in building leaner muscles that are not easily burned away during the performance. People might wonder as to how vegans can meet this protein requirement without the addition of meats and eggs to their diet.

The answer lies in oatmeal, as they can easily replace these ingredients and increase body proteins by a large margin. Just ½ a cup of cooked oats can contain 7 to 9 grams of proteins, which is ideal for athletes. Dry oats are often added to pre-post workout shakes in order to capitalize on their protein content.

Iron

An athlete's body requires a good dose of iron, as it binds with oxygen and circulates throughout the body. A cup of cooked oats is capable of providing you with 18% of the minimum requirement thereby making it a must have in the mornings.

Beta glucans

No athlete's diet will be complete without the addition of foods that are rich in beta glucans. These help in draining cholesterol from the bloodstream and provide the body with ample soluble fibers. You will have the chance to develop a leaner waistline through the consumption of oatmeal on a regular basis.

As a vegan, you can prepare oats using water or substitute milk with almond or soymilk.

3) LEAFY GREENS (KALE AND SPINACH)

Leafy green vegetables are loaded with multiple vitamins that are required to maintain a healthy body. There are several types of leafy green vegetables that one can choose from, but kale and spinach take top billing for the amazing health benefits that they provide. Some of these benefits are as follows.

- Kale

Nutrients

Kale is rich in many essential nutrients including iron, Vitamins A, C and K. All of these help in increasing your body's capacity in recovering from muscle soreness. It also contains the highest amount of lutein, which is a potent antioxidant. Kale assists in enhancing cell repair and ensures that your body has the chance to fully recover after each session.

Cholesterol

It is obvious that no athlete will be able to resist the temptation of digging into some of their favorite snacks. This includes potato chips and wafers that athletes tend to eat, feeling guilty. However, one great substitute for this can be baked kale chips. They taste great and ensure that you do not subject yourself to unnecessary calories and cholesterol. In fact, kale is known to cut down on the level of cholesterol in your blood stream thereby making it the best snacking option for vegan athletes.

- Spinach

Calories

Spinach is low in calorie content. Spinach can be quite filling without the addition of unwanted calories. Just a quick blitz in the blender and you are left with a healthy juice sure to increase your nutrition through several folds.

Energy

Spinach is said to contain nitrates that contribute toward increasing cellular efficiency. You will feel energetic before and after a workout and have enough energy to carry on without feeling too tired.

Bones

It is crucial for athletes, especially women athletes, to pay keen attention to their bone health. Excessive pressure on bones during workout and performance can weaken them and lead to bone deficiencies. One good way of dealing with this is through the incorporation of spinach in your day-to-day diet. Spinach contains vitamin K in abundance, which is required to maintain strong bones. It also contains calcium that can further improve bone health.

Fiber

Fiber is required to digest food and maintain a clean stomach. Spinach can provide you with a good dose of fiber. Just a cup of spinach juice will leave you with 3 to 4 grams of fiber.

Apart from kale and spinach, you can also consume arugula, chard, collard greens, curly endive and tatsoi.

4) NUTS (WALNUTS AND ALMONDS)

Walnuts are nutritional powerhouses designed to keep your body strong and healthy. Just a handful of walnuts are enough to increase your overall health and make you a better athlete.

• Walnuts

Here is why walnuts make for an athlete's best friend.

Amino acid

Amino acids are required for the upkeep of cells and muscles. In fact, it forms a large part of our body's cell structure. Walnuts contain an amino acid known as L-arginine, which is required to maintain muscle health. This amino acid converts to nitric oxide, a compound that causes blood vessels to dilate. This improves blood flow to the various muscles and reduces the risk of tearing.

Omega 3 fatty acids

Walnuts consist of omega 3 fatty acids that are required to maintain heart health. It reduces inflammation and helps with the conversion of fat to energy. In fact, walnuts are regarded as the number 1 vegan substitute for fish oils, as they can contain just as much fatty acids. Omega 3 acids are also said to enhance exercise performance. You will be able to exercise for longer hours.

Nutrients

Walnuts are rich in multiple nutrients including B vitamins and zinc. These aid in keeping the immune system healthy. You will fall sick less often and be able to perform better.

• Almonds

Almonds are the second best nuts to add to your diet. They are just as nutritious as walnuts, if not more.

Here is what makes almonds good for your body.

Calcium

Almonds contain a high dose of calcium that is required to maintain strong bones. Just by nibbling on a few almonds you will be able to increase the calcium content in your bones and prevent them from drawing from your bloodstream.

Fiber

The fiber content in almonds is extremely high, making it ideal for athletes. Fiber is not digested by the body and tricks it into working hard to digest it. This causes the body to up its metabolism and assists with improving digestion.

Protein

Almonds have a fair amount of proteins that can contribute to your daily requirement. Munching on a few before and after your workout session can leave you energetic and help your muscles recover faster.

Magnesium

Magnesium is an important component of the body and especially required by athletes to remain healthy. It helps in enhancing the release of testosterone and controlling cortisol thereby enabling better performance.

Both walnuts and almonds can be added to smoothies or toasted and sprinkled over salads.

5) SWEET POTATOES

The next vegan super food to add to your diet is sweet potatoes. Here is why you should make it a big part of your daily diet.

Energy

Sweet potatoes provide you with truckloads of energy. Regardless of the sport you play, you are sure to experience a marked difference in your energy levels through the consumption of sweet potatoes. The energy will be consistent and last throughout the day.

Vitamin A

Sweet potatoes are loaded with vitamin A and in fact, can meet 100% of your daily requirement. Vitamin A is an essential antioxidant that is needed to boost your immune system. It checks infections and keeps you healthy from the inside out.

Inflammation

Sweet potatoes control inflammation to a large extent. Athletes run the risk of suffering from muscle inflammation. The best way to deal with this is through the consumption of sweet potatoes. Not only do they control inflammation but also help in reducing non-contact injuries.

Glycemic index

High glycemic foods are those that spike up blood sugar levels in your body. Although this might seem ideal for an athlete, it is important to avoid such foods as much as possible as it can lead to the development of diabetes type 2. Sweet potatoes happen to curb the release of sugars and control insulin levels in the bloodstream.

Complex carbs

Sweet potatoes consist of a set of complex carbs that are not easily digested by the body. This makes it an ideal food to consume post workout, as the body will continue to burn fat. It also helps in adding back some of the lost energy, so that you have enough left to carry out the remaining chores.

Magnesium and potassium

Sweet potatoes contain magnesium and potassium, both of which help in controlling muscle spasms. They also help in controlling cramps and improve muscle function. Any injured muscles will recover faster thereby enhancing your performance drive.

6) SEEDS (CHIA AND SESAME SEEDS)

• Chia seeds

Chia seeds are very nutritious and can provide athletes with sustained energy. They are favorites among runners and gym goers. Here are some of its health benefits.

Dehydration

Chia seeds have the capacity of holding almost 30 times their weight in water and can, therefore, provide the body with consistent hydration. They are ideal for athletes and exercisers who work out in humid climates and require more hydration than others.

Joint aches

Rich in omega 3 fatty acids, Chia seeds help in creating a lubricating barrier between joints.

This helps in reducing inflammation and facilitates movement. These oils also help in controlling hyperactivity and hypertension.

Weight loss

Since these seeds absorb far more water than their capacity, they can be consumed to feel fuller for longer. Just a handful will do the job and you do not have to worry about feeling puckish in between meals.

Recovery

The amino acids found in Chia seeds can help in accelerating recovery time. It can decrease the time taken by your muscles to recover from soreness. They are therefore best eaten as soon as you step out of the gym, or finish your exercise routine. A cup of Chia seeds can leave you with 10 grams of fiber.

• <u>Sesame seeds</u>

Sesame seeds are the next best seeds to add to your diet. They might be tiny but are loaded with nutrition. Here are some of the health benefits provided by sesame seeds.

Calcium

Sesame seeds are a storehouse of calcium. Calcium is important for all athletes as it can easily deplete during workouts. 30 grams of sesame seeds can provide the body with 350 grams of calcium. This makes for nearly 40% of the daily requirement.

Iron

Iron is required by the body to produce hemoglobin that transports oxygen to the different muscle tissues. 30 grams of sesame seeds can provide you with 5 grams of iron, which happens to be 60% of the daily requirement for men.

Zinc

As per studies, athletes and bodybuilders have a high risk of developing zinc deficiency. This can lead to fatigue, reduced endurance and brain fog. Sesame seeds, being rich in zinc content, can solve this problem once and for all. You will feel energetic and experience enhanced performance.

As you can see, chewing on a few chia and sesame seeds on a day-to-day basis can help you enhance your athletic performance.

7) BANANA

Rounding up the list of superfoods is the humble banana. Bananas are an athlete's ideal food as they are loaded with vital nutrients. They are as follows.

Potassium

Bananas are rich in potassium content. A single banana has 450 mg of potassium, which makes for 14% of your daily requirement. Potassium helps in controlling blood sugar levels and can enhance heart function. Potassium can protect your heart by curbing high blood pressure. Athletes have the tendency of feeling dehydrated quite often. The best solution is to consume a banana as it acts as an electrolyte and balances body fluids.

Potassium can also greatly reduce the occurrence of muscle cramps and contribute towards the development of stronger, leaner muscles.

Carbohydrates

A single banana can contain 30 grams of carbohydrates, thereby making it ideal for athletes. Consuming half a banana before a workout session will ensure that you have enough energy to last you through the day. You can follow up your workout with another half in order to add back some of the lost energy. As per experiments conducted on gymnasts, bananas helped in improving their reflexes. Those who consumed a banana before their balance beam routines were able to stave off falls.

Vitamin C

A single banana can provide you with 15% of your daily vitamin C requirement. Vitamin C is an important component required to strengthen muscles, ligaments and tendons. It is also responsible for increasing immunity and providing fast relief from wounds- acquired while working out. It is also responsible for synthesizing adrenaline required to carry out day-to-day exercise routines.

Bananas are easily available and quite cheap. You can consume half a large banana before your workout, and one after.

CONCLUSION

Superfoods are great for your body because of their nutrition content. It will do wonders for your health and energy. Not just that, it will also speed up your workout recovery time! At the same time, you can strengthen your mind as well as build lean muscle.

When it comes to working out, endurance, strength and recovery are the most important parts of the puzzle. I hope you develop the body of your dream and excel in your sport. Good luck!

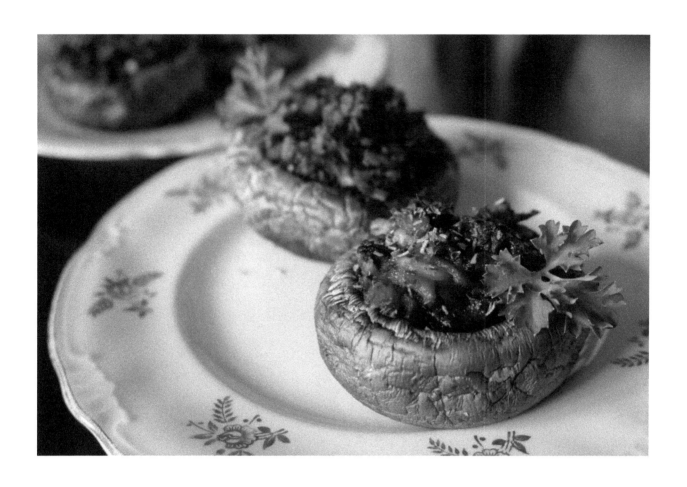

72 DELICIOUS RECIPES

Vegan Refried Beans

Ingredients

1 tablespoon olive oil
1 onion, diced
1 (15 ounce) can pinto beans, drained
3 tablespoons tomato paste
chili powder to taste
1 cup vegetable broth

Directions

Heat oil in a medium skillet over medium heat. Saute onions until tender. Stir in beans, tomato paste, chili powder and vegetable broth. Cook 5 minutes, or until stock has reduced. Mash with a potato masher.

Vegan Carrot Soup

Ingredients

1 tablespoon vegetable oil
1 large onion, diced
3 cloves garlic, minced
4 large carrots, sliced
5 new potatoes, quartered
2 cups vegetable broth
2 teaspoons grated fresh ginger
1 teaspoon curry powder
salt and pepper to taste

Directions

Heat oil in a soup pot over medium heat. Add onion and garlic, and cook stirring often until onion is translucent. Add carrots and potatoes, and cook for just a few minutes to allow the carrots to sweat out some of their juices.

Pour the vegetable broth into the pot, and season with ginger, curry powder, salt and pepper. Bring to a boil, then reduce heat to low. Simmer for 15 to 20 minutes, until carrots are tender.

Puree soup in small batches using a food processor or blender, or if you have an immersion blender, it can be done in the soup pot. Reheat soup if necessary, and serve.

Vegan Pancakes

Ingredients

1 1/4 cups all-purpose flour
2 tablespoons white sugar
2 teaspoons baking powder
1/2 teaspoon salt
1 1/4 cups water
1 tablespoon oil

Directions

Sift the flour, sugar, baking powder, and salt into a large bowl. Whisk the water and oil together in a small bowl. Make a well in the center of the dry ingredients, and pour in the wet. Stir just until blended; mixture will be lumpy.

Heat a lightly oiled griddle over medium-high heat. Drop batter by large spoonfuls onto the griddle, and cook until bubbles form and the edges are dry. Flip, and cook until browned on the other side. Repeat with remaining batter.

Vegan Casserole

Ingredients

5 russet potatoes, peeled
1 clove crushed garlic
1 stalk celery, chopped
1 bunch fresh parsley, chopped
8 whole black peppercorns
1 onion, chopped
1 bay leaf
1 tablespoon light miso paste
1 tablespoon olive oil

1 tablespoon olive oil
3/4 cup diced red onion
1 clove garlic, minced
1/2 pound fresh mushrooms, sliced
1 pound firm tofu, crumbled
4 tablespoons hickory flavored barbecue sauce
1 tablespoon nutritional yeast (optional)
1 tablespoon vegetarian chicken flavored gravy mix
1 teaspoon paprika
1 tablespoon tamari
1 cup fresh corn kernels
1 cup chopped spinach

2 tablespoons olive oil
1/8 cup whole wheat pastry flour
2 teaspoons nutritional yeast (optional)
1 tablespoon vegetarian chicken flavored gravy mix
1 cube vegetable bouillon

Directions

Preheat oven to 400 degrees F (200 degrees C).

Peel and quarter potatoes. Place in a medium or large size pot with water to cover. Add garlic, celery, parsley, peppercorns, onion, and bay leaf. Bring to a boil, cover, and simmer over medium-low heat for 15 to 20 minutes or until potatoes are very tender.

To Make Filling: While potatoes are cooking, in a large skillet heat 1 tablespoon oil and saute onion and garlic. Saute for 1 minute over medium heat, then add mushrooms and saute for 2 minutes. Crumble tofu in chunks into the skillet and saute briefly, mixing well. Stir in barbecue sauce, yeast, gravy mix, thyme, paprika, and tamari. Mix well and saute, stirring frequently, for 20 minutes over medium heat.

Transfer potatoes from water to a large bowl, reserving 3 1/2 cups of the remaining stock. Add miso, oil, and 3/4 to 1 cup of the potato stock to the potatoes a little at a time, mashing potatoes as you add the stock. Add only enough water to moisten potatoes adequately. Do not over moisten, this potato mixture will be the crust covering of the casserole.

Add corn and spinach to filling mixture and mix well. Spoon filling into an oiled, shallow ovenproof casserole dish. Pat down with back of a large spoon. Spread potato crust evenly over filling, smoothing top with a spoon or spatula. Dust evenly with paprika. Bake for 30 to 40 minutes, or until crust is golden.

While casserole bakes, prepare gravy. Heat oil in a large frying pan. Add flour and yeast, stir with a whisk over medium heat to form a paste. Slowly stir in 2 1/2 cups of reserved potato water, whisking as you stir to allow gravy to thicken. Stir in instant gravy mix and continue whisking until gravy is thick and smooth; add additional potato water, if necessary. Serve casserole with crust on the bottom and filling on top. Spoon gravy over top.

Harvest Vegan Nut Roast

Ingredients

1/2 cup chopped celery
2 onions, chopped
3/4 cup walnuts
3/4 cup pecan or sunflower meal
2 1/2 cups soy milk
1 teaspoon dried basil
1 teaspoon dried oregano
3 cups bread crumbs
salt and pepper to taste

Directions

Preheat oven to 350 degrees F (175 degrees C). Lightly oil a loaf pan.

In a medium size frying pan, saute the chopped celery and the onion in 3 teaspoons water until cooked.

In a large mixing bowl combine the celery and onion with walnuts, pecan or sunflower meal, soy milk, basil, oregano, bread crumbs, salt and pepper to taste; mix well. Place mixture in the prepared loaf pan.

Bake for 60 to 90 minutes; until the loaf is cooked through.

Vegan Davy Crockett Bars

Ingredients

2 cups all-purpose flour
1 cup white sugar
1 teaspoon salt
1 teaspoon baking powder
1 teaspoon baking soda
1 cup brown sugar
2 cups quick cooking oats
1 cup vegan chocolate chips
1 teaspoon vanilla extract
3/4 cup vegetable oil

Directions

Preheat an oven to 350 degrees F (175 degrees C).

Mix flour, sugar, salt, baking powder, and baking soda together in a large bowl. Stir in brown sugar, oats, and chocolate chips. In a separate bowl, combine oil and vanilla extract; stir into flour mixture. Press dough into a 15x10 inch jelly roll pan.

Bake in the preheated oven until lightly brown, about 15 minutes. Cool before cutting into bars.

Creamy Vegan Corn Chowder

Ingredients

2 tablespoons olive oil
1 small onion, chopped
1 cup celery, chopped
1 cup carrots, chopped
1 clove garlic, minced
2 1/2 cups water
2 cubes vegetable bouillon
2 cups corn
2 cups soy milk
1 tablespoon flour
1 teaspoon dried parsley
1 teaspoon garlic powder
1 teaspoon salt
1 teaspoon pepper

Directions

Heat oil in a large skillet over medium heat. Stir in onions and celery; cook until just slightly golden. Stir in carrots and garlic; cook until garlic is slightly golden.

Meanwhile, bring water to a boil over high heat. Stir in bouillon, and reduce heat to medium. When bouillon cubes have dissolved, add corn and the vegetables from the skillet. Cook until vegetables are tender. Add water, if necessary. Reduce heat to low, and pour in 1 cup soy milk. Stir soup well, then stir in remaining 1 cup soy milk. Quickly whisk in flour. Stir in parsley, garlic powder, salt, and pepper. Cook, stirring constantly, until chowder thickens, about 15 to 20 minutes.

'Dark Night' Vegan Chocolate Mousse

Ingredients

1 (16 ounce) package silken tofu, drained
3/4 cup Stevia Extract In The Raw® Cup For Cup
1 teaspoon pure vanilla extract
1 tablespoon light agave syrup
1/4 cup soy milk
1/2 cup unsweetened cocoa powder
2 tablespoons carob powder
Mint leaves

Directions

Place tofu, Stevia Extract In The Raw and vanilla in a food processor or blender. Process until well blended. Add remaining ingredients and process until mixture is fully blended.

Pour into small dessert cups or espresso cups. Chill for at least 2 hours. Garnish with fresh mint leaves just before serving.

Vegan Peanut Butter Fudge

Ingredients

2 cups packed brown sugar
1/8 teaspoon salt
3/4 cup soy milk
2 tablespoons light corn syrup
4 tablespoons peanut butter
1 teaspoon vanilla extract

Directions

Lightly grease one 9x5x2 inch pan.

In a 2-quart pot over very low heat, mix together the brown sugar, salt, soy milk, corn syrup, peanut butter and vanilla. Cook until hot and brown sugar is dissolved.

Quickly pour into pan and refrigerate. Cut into squares and store in semi-airtight container in refrigerator.

Creamy Vegan Hot Cocoa

Ingredients

3 tablespoons canned coconut milk
1/2 teaspoon vanilla extract
3 tablespoons white sugar
4 1/2 teaspoons cocoa powder
1 dash ground cinnamon
1 cup boiling water

Directions

Stir together coconut milk, vanilla extract, sugar, cocoa powder, and cinnamon in a large mug. Add boiling water and stir until the sugar has dissolved.

Vegan Apple Carrot Muffins

Ingredients

1 cup brown sugar
1/2 cup white sugar
2 1/2 cups all-purpose flour
4 teaspoons baking soda
1 teaspoon baking powder
4 teaspoons ground cinnamon
2 teaspoons salt
2 cups finely grated carrots
2 large apples - peeled, cored and shredded
6 teaspoons egg replacer (dry)
1 1/4 cups applesauce
1/4 cup vegetable oil

Directions

Preheat oven to 375 degrees F (190 degrees C). Grease muffin cups or line with paper muffin liners.

In a large bowl combine brown sugar, white sugar, flour, baking soda, baking powder, cinnamon and salt. Stir in carrot and apple; mix well.

In a small bowl whisk together egg substitute, applesauce and oil. Stir into dry ingredients.

Spoon batter into prepared pans.

Bake in preheated oven for 20 minutes. Let muffins cool in pan for 5 minutes before removing from pans to cool completely.

Vegan Lentil, Kale, and Red Onion Pasta

Ingredients

2 1/2 cups vegetable broth
3/4 cup dry lentils
1/2 teaspoon salt
1 bay leaf

1/4 cup olive oil
1 large red onion, chopped
1 teaspoon chopped fresh thyme
1/2 teaspoon chopped fresh oregano
1/2 teaspoon salt
1/2 teaspoon black pepper
8 ounces vegan sausage, cut into 1/4 inch slices (optional)

1 bunch kale, stems removed and leaves coarsely chopped
1 (12 ounce) package rotini pasta
2 tablespoons nutritional yeast (optional)

Directions

Bring the vegetable broth, lentils, 1/2 teaspoon of salt, and bay leaf to a boil in a saucepan over high heat. Reduce heat to medium-low, cover, and cook until the lentils are tender, about 20 minutes. Add additional broth if needed to keep the lentils moist. Discard the bay leaf once done.

As the lentils simmer, heat the olive oil in a skillet over medium-high heat. Stir in the onion, thyme, oregano, 1/2 teaspoon of salt, and pepper. Cook and stir for 1 minute, then add the sausage. Reduce the heat to medium-low, and cook until the onion has softened, about 10 minutes.

Meanwhile, bring a large pot of lightly salted water to a boil over high heat. Add the kale and rotini pasta. Cook until the rotini is al dente, about 8 minutes. Remove some of the cooking water, and set aside. Drain the pasta, then return to the pot, and stir in the lentils, and onion mixture. Use the reserved cooking liquid to adjust the moistness of the dish to your liking. Sprinkle with nutritional yeast to serve.

Vegan Granola

Ingredients

cooking spray
3 cups rolled oats
2/3 cup wheat germ
1/2 cup slivered almonds
1 pinch ground nutmeg
1 1/2 teaspoons ground cinnamon
1/2 cup apple juice
1/2 cup molasses
1 teaspoon vanilla extract
1 cup dried mixed fruit
1 cup quartered dried apricots

Directions

Preheat oven to 350 degrees F (175 degrees C). Prepare two cookie sheets with cooking spray.

In a large bowl, combine oats, wheat germ, almonds, cinnamon and nutmeg. In a separate bowl, mix apple juice, molasses and extract. Pour the wet ingredients into the dry ingredients, stirring to coat. Spread mixture onto baking sheets.

Bake for 30 minutes in preheated oven, stirring mixture every 10 to 15 minutes, or until granola has a golden brown color. Let cool. Stir in dried fruit. Store in an airtight container.

Vegan Baked Oatmeal Patties

Ingredients

4 cups water
4 cups quick cooking oats
1/2 onion, chopped
1/3 cup vegetable oil
1/2 cup spaghetti sauce
1/2 cup chopped pecans
1/4 cup nutritional yeast
2 teaspoons garlic powder
1 teaspoon dried basil
2 teaspoons onion powder
1 teaspoon ground coriander
1 teaspoon sage
1 teaspoon active dry yeast

Directions

Preheat oven to 350 degrees F (175 degrees C). Grease a baking sheet.

Bring water to a boil and stir in oatmeal. Cover and reduce heat to low. Cook 5 to 10 minutes, or until the oats are cooked and all the water has been absorbed. Remove from heat and let stand for 5 minutes.

To the oatmeal add onion, oil, spaghetti sauce, pecans, nutritional yeast, garlic powder, basil, onion powder, coriander, sage and active yeast. Mix well and form into patties. Place on prepared baking sheet.

Bake for 15 minutes. Turn patties over and bake another 15 minutes.

Vegan Black Bean Soup

Ingredients

1 tablespoon olive oil
1 large onion, chopped
1 stalk celery, chopped
2 carrots, chopped
4 cloves garlic, chopped
2 tablespoons chili powder
1 tablespoon ground cumin
1 pinch black pepper
4 cups vegetable broth
4 (15 ounce) cans black beans
1 (15 ounce) can whole kernel corn
1 (14.5 ounce) can crushed tomatoes

Directions

Heat oil in a large pot over medium-high heat. Saute onion, celery, carrots and garlic for 5 minutes. Season with chili powder, cumin, and black pepper; cook for 1 minute. Stir in vegetable broth, 2 cans of beans, and corn. Bring to a boil.

Meanwhile, in a food processor or blender, process remaining 2 cans beans and tomatoes until smooth. Stir into boiling soup mixture, reduce heat to medium, and simmer for 15 minutes.

Vegan Taco Chili

Ingredients

1 tablespoon olive oil
1 pound sliced fresh mushrooms
2 cloves garlic, minced
1 small onion, finely chopped
2 stalks celery, chopped
1 (29 ounce) can tomato sauce
1 (6 ounce) can tomato paste
3 (15 ounce) cans kidney beans
1 (11 ounce) can Mexican-style corn

Directions

Heat the oil in a large skillet. Sautee the mushrooms, garlic, onion and celery until tender. Transfer them to a stock pot or slow cooker. Stir in the tomato sauce, tomato paste, beans and Mexican-style corn. Cook for at least an hour to blend the flavors.

Easy Vegan Whole Grain Pancakes

Ingredients

1/2 cup whole wheat flour
1/2 cup rye flour
1 tablespoon soy flour
1 tablespoon white sugar
1 1/2 teaspoons baking powder
1/8 teaspoon salt
1/8 teaspoon ground cinnamon
(optional)
1/2 teaspoon vanilla extract
(optional)
1/2 cup water
1/2 cup soy milk
1/4 cup chopped pecans

Directions

In a medium bowl, stir together the whole wheat flour, rye flour, soy flour, sugar, baking powder, salt and cinnamon. Make a well in the center, and pour in the vanilla, water and soy milk. Mix until all of the dry ingredients have been absorbed, then stir in the pecans.

Heat a large skillet or griddle iron over medium heat, and coat with cooking spray. Pour about 1/3 cup of batter onto the hot surface, and spread out to 1/4 inch thickness. Cook until bubbles appear on the surface, then flip and brown on the other side. Serve warm.

Vegan Stew

Ingredients

1 onion, chopped
3 carrots, chopped
3 potatoes, chopped
1 parsnip, chopped
1 turnip, chopped
1/4 cup uncooked white rice
1 teaspoon ground black pepper
1 teaspoon ground cumin
1 teaspoon salt
2 1/2 cups water

Directions

In a large pot over medium-high heat, combine onion, carrots, potatoes, parsnip, turnip, rice, pepper, cumin, salt and water. Boil until vegetables are tender, about 30 minutes, adding more water if necessary.

Vegan Crepes

Ingredients

1/2 cup soy milk
1/2 cup water
1/4 cup melted soy margarine
1 tablespoon turbinado sugar
2 tablespoons maple syrup
1 cup unbleached all-purpose flour
1/4 teaspoon salt

Directions

In a large mixing bowl, blend soy milk, water, 1/4 cup margarine, sugar, syrup, flour, and salt. Cover and chill the mixture for 2 hours.

Lightly grease a 5 to 6 inch skillet with some soy margarine. Heat the skillet until hot. Pour approximately 3 tablespoons batter into the skillet. Swirl to make the batter cover the skillet's bottom. Cook until golden, flip and cook on opposite side.

Vegan Chocolate Cake

Ingredients

1 1/2 cups all-purpose flour
1 cup white sugar
1/4 cup cocoa powder
1 teaspoon baking soda
1/2 teaspoon salt
1/3 cup vegetable oil
1 teaspoon vanilla extract
1 teaspoon distilled white vinegar
1 cup water

Directions

Preheat oven to 350 degrees F (175 degrees C). Lightly grease one 9x5 inch loaf pan.

Sift together the flour, sugar, cocoa, baking soda and salt. Add the oil, vanilla, vinegar and water. Mix together until smooth.

Pour into prepared pan and bake at 350 degrees F (175 degrees C) for 45 minutes. Remove from oven and allow to cool.

Cyclops Cookies (Vegan)

Ingredients

2 cups all-purpose flour
1/4 teaspoon ground cinnamon
1/4 cup shortening
1/4 cup margarine
3/4 cup confectioners' sugar
1 cup chopped walnuts
1 cup semisweet chocolate chips

Directions

Mix together the flour and cinnamon. In separate large bowl cream together shortening, margarine and powdered sugar. Gradually add in the flour/cinnamon mixture. Fold in the chopped nuts.

Roll out on floured surface to 1/4 inch thickness and cut out cookies with a 2 inch round cookie cutter. Place 1 inch apart on ungreased cookie sheet.

Put one single chocolate chip in the center of each cookie. Bake 8 -10 minutes at 400 degrees F (205 degrees C) until lightly colored. Cool on wire racks.

Ingredients

2 tablespoons olive oil
1 1/2 cups chopped onion
3 tablespoons minced garlic
4 (14.5 ounce) cans stewed tomatoes
1/3 cup tomato paste
1/2 cup chopped fresh basil
1/2 cup chopped parsley
1 teaspoon salt
1 teaspoon ground black pepper

1 (16 ounce) package lasagna noodles

2 pounds firm tofu
2 tablespoons minced garlic
1/4 cup chopped fresh basil
1/4 cup chopped parsley
1/2 teaspoon salt
ground black pepper to taste
3 (10 ounce) packages frozen chopped spinach, thawed and drained

Directions

Make the sauce: In a large, heavy saucepan, over medium heat, heat the olive oil. Place the onions in the saucepan and saute them until they are soft, about 5 minutes. Add the garlic; cook 5 minutes more.

Place the tomatoes, tomato paste, basil and parsley in the saucepan. Stir well, turn the heat to low and let the sauce simmer covered for 1 hour. Add the salt and pepper.

While the sauce is cooking bring a large kettle of salted water to a boil. Boil the lasagna noodles for 9 minutes, then drain and rinse well.

Preheat the oven to 400 degrees F (200 degrees C).

Place the tofu blocks in a large bowl. Add the garlic, basil and parsley. Add the salt and pepper, and mash all the ingredients together by squeezing pieces of tofu through your fingers. Mix well.

Assemble the lasagna: Spread 1 cup of the tomato sauce in the bottom of a 9x13 inch casserole pan. Arrange a single layer of lasagna noodles, sprinkle one-third of the tofu mixture over the noodles. Distribute the spinach evenly over the tofu. Next ladle 1 1/2 cups tomato sauce over the tofu, and top it with another layer of the noodles. Then sprinkle another 1/3 of the tofu mixture over the noodles, top the tofu with 1 1/2 cups tomato sauce, and place a final layer of noodles over the tomato sauce. Finally, top the noodles with the final 1/3 of the tofu, and spread the remaining tomato sauce over everything.

Cover the pan with foil and bake the lasagna for 30 minutes. Serve hot and enjoy.

Easy Vegan Peanut Butter Fudge

Ingredients

3/4 cup vegan margarine
1 cup peanut butter
3 2/3 cups confectioners' sugar

Directions

Lightly grease a 9x9 inch baking dish.

In a saucepan over low heat, melt margarine. Remove from heat and stir in peanut butter until smooth. Stir in confectioners' sugar, a little at a time, until well blended. Pat into prepared pan and chill until firm. Cut into squares.

Yummy Vegan Chocolate Pudding

Ingredients

2 tablespoons cornstarch
1 cup soy milk
1 cup soy creamer
1/2 cup white sugar
3 tablespoons egg replacer (dry)
3 ounces semisweet chocolate, chopped
2 teaspoons vanilla extract

Directions

In a medium saucepan combine cornstarch, soy milk and soy creamer; stir to dissolve cornstarch. Place on medium heat and stir in sugar. Cook, whisking frequently, until mixture comes to a low boil; remove from heat.

In a small bowl whisk egg replacer with 1/4 cup of hot milk mixture; return to pan with remaining milk mixture. Cook over medium heat for 3 to 4 minutes, until thick, but not boiling.

Place the chocolate in a medium bowl and pour in the hot milk mixture. Let stand for 30 seconds, then stir until melted and smooth. Cool for 10 to 15 minutes, then stir in vanilla.

Pour into ramekins or custard cups. Cover with plastic wrap and let cool at room temperature. Refrigerate for 3 hours, or overnight before serving.

Fluffy Vegan Pancakes

Ingredients

1 1/4 cups all-purpose flour
1 tablespoon baking powder
1/2 teaspoon fine sea salt
1/4 cup pureed extra-firm tofu
1 cup soy milk
1 tablespoon canola oil
1/2 cup water

Directions

Whisk together the flour, baking powder, and sea salt; set aside.

Whisk together the tofu, soy milk, canola oil, and water. Gradually whisk the flour mixture into the tofu mixture, making sure to beat out all lumps between additions.

Heat a lightly oiled griddle over medium-high heat. Drop batter by large spoonfuls onto the griddle, and cook until lightly browned on the bottom. Flip, and cook until lightly browned on the other side. Repeat with remaining batter.

Val and Jess's Vegan Avocado Dip

Ingredients

2 avocados - peeled, pitted and diced
1 (19 ounce) can black beans, drained and rinsed
1 (11 ounce) can whole kernel corn, drained
1 medium onion, minced
3/4 cup salsa
1 tablespoon chopped fresh cilantro
1 tablespoon lemon juice
2 tablespoons chili powder
salt and pepper to taste

Directions

In a bowl, mix the avocados, black beans, corn, onion, salsa, cilantro, and lemon juice. Season with chili powder, salt, and pepper.

Vegan Curried Rice

Ingredients

2 tablespoons olive oil
1 tablespoon minced garlic
black pepper to taste
1 tablespoon ground cumin, or to taste
1 tablespoon ground curry powder, or to taste
1 tablespoon chili powder, or to taste
1 cube vegetable bouillon
1 cup water
1 tablespoon soy sauce
1 cup uncooked white rice

Directions

Heat olive oil in a medium saucepan over low heat. Sweat the garlic; when the garlic becomes aromatic, slowly stir in pepper, cumin, curry powder and chili powder. When spices begin to fry and become fragrant, stir in the bouillon cube and a little water.

Increase heat to high and add the rest of the water and the soy sauce. Just before the mixture comes to a boil, stir in rice. Bring to a rolling boil; reduce heat to low, cover, and simmer 15 to 20 minutes, or until all liquid is absorbed.

Remove from heat and let stand 5 minutes.

Vegan-Friendly Falafel

Ingredients

1 pound dry garbanzo beans
1 onion, quartered
1 potato, peeled and quartered
4 cloves garlic, minced
1/2 cup cilantro leaves, chopped
1 teaspoon ground coriander
1 teaspoon ground cumin
2 teaspoons salt
1/2 teaspoon ground black pepper
1/2 teaspoon cayenne pepper
2 teaspoons fresh lemon juice
1 tablespoon olive oil
1 tablespoon all-purpose flour
2 teaspoons baking soda
2 cups canola oil

Directions

Rinse the garbanzo beans under cold water and discard any bad ones. Place in a large pot, and cover with water. Let soak 24 hours, and rinse again.

Place the garbanzo beans, onion, and potato in the bowl of a food processor. Cover, and process until finely chopped. Leaving about 1 cup of the garbanzo bean mixture in the food processor bowl, pour the rest into a mixing bowl. Add the garlic, cilantro, coriander, cumin, salt, pepper, and cayenne pepper to the garbanzo bean mixture in the food processor bowl; process on low to blend thoroughly. Return the reserved garbanzo bean mixture to the food processor bowl, and add the lemon juice, and olive oil; process on low into a coarse meal. Cover, and refrigerate 2 hours.

Stir the baking soda into the garbanzo bean mixture until evenly blended. Using damp hands, form the mixture into 1 1/2 inch diameter balls.

Pour the canola oil into a wok 1 to 2 inches deep, and heat over medium-high heat. Cook the falafel balls, turning so all sides are evenly browned, about 5 minutes. Remove falafel from oil, and drain on paper towels. Repeat to cook remaining falafel balls.

Simple Vegan Icing

Ingredients

1/2 cup vegetable shortening
4 cups confectioners' sugar
5 tablespoons soy milk
1/4 teaspoon vanilla extract

Directions

Beat the shortening and confectioners' sugar together until the shortening has been incorporated, and the mixture is clumpy. Pour in the soy milk and vanilla extract; beat until smooth.

Penne with Vegan Arrabbiata Sauce

Ingredients

1 cup extra virgin olive oil
7 cloves garlic, minced
7 (28 ounce) cans crushed tomatoes
2 1/2 teaspoons crushed red pepper flakes
2 bay leaves
10 leaves fresh basil

Directions

Bring a large pot of lightly salted water to a boil. Add pasta and cook for 8 to 10 minutes or until al dente; drain.

Heat olive oil, and cook garlic just until softened. Add remaining ingredients. Simmer over low heat and cook at least 3 hours.

Add the cooked penne pasta and let sit at least 5 minutes before stirring and serving. Sprinkle with 1/2 cup grated Romano or parmesan cheese, if desired.

Kingman's Vegan Zucchini Bread

Ingredients

3 cups all-purpose flour
3 tablespoons flax seeds (optional)
1 teaspoon salt
1 teaspoon baking soda
2 teaspoons ground cinnamon
1/2 teaspoon baking powder
1/2 teaspoon arrowroot powder (optional)
1 cup unsweetened applesauce
1 cup white sugar
1 cup packed brown sugar
3/4 cup vegetable oil
2 teaspoons vanilla extract
2 1/2 cups shredded zucchini

Directions

Preheat oven to 325 degrees F (165 degrees C). Grease and flour two 9x5 inch loaf pans. Whisk together the flour, flax seeds, salt, baking soda, cinnamon, baking powder, and arrowroot in a bowl until evenly blended; set aside.

Whisk together the applesauce, white sugar, brown sugar, vegetable oil, and vanilla extract in a bowl until smooth. Fold in the flour mixture and shredded zucchini until moistened. Divide the batter between the prepared loaf pans.

Bake in the preheated oven until a toothpick inserted into the center comes out clean, about 70 minutes. Cool in the pans for 10 minutes before removing to cool completely on a wire rack.

Vegan Red Lentil Soup

Ingredients

1 tablespoon peanut oil
1 small onion, chopped
1 tablespoon minced fresh ginger root
1 clove garlic, chopped
1 pinch fenugreek seeds
1 cup dry red lentils
1 cup butternut squash - peeled, seeded, and cubed
1/3 cup finely chopped fresh cilantro
2 cups water
1/2 (14 ounce) can coconut milk
2 tablespoons tomato paste
1 teaspoon curry powder
1 pinch cayenne pepper
1 pinch ground nutmeg
salt and pepper to taste

Directions

Heat the oil in a large pot over medium heat, and cook the onion, ginger, garlic, and fenugreek until onion is tender.

Mix the lentils, squash, and cilantro into the pot. Stir in the water, coconut milk, and tomato paste. Season with curry powder, cayenne pepper, nutmeg, salt, and pepper. Bring to a boil, reduce heat to low, and simmer 30 minutes, or until lentils and squash are tender.

Vegan Lemon Poppy Scones

Ingredients

2 cups all-purpose flour
3/4 cup white sugar
4 teaspoons baking powder
1/2 teaspoon salt
3/4 cup margarine
1 lemon, zested and juiced
2 tablespoons poppy seeds
1/2 cup soy milk
1/2 cup water

Directions

Preheat the oven to 400 degrees F (200 degrees C). Grease a baking sheet.

Sift the flour, sugar, baking powder and salt into a large bowl. Cut in margarine until the mixture is the consistency of large grains of sand. I like to use my hands to rub the margarine into the flour. Stir in poppy seeds, lemon zest and lemon juice. Combine the soy milk and water, and gradually stir into the dry ingredients until the batter is moistened, but still thick like biscuit dough. You may not need all of the liquid.

Spoon 1/4 cup sized plops of batter onto the greased baking sheet so they are about 3 inches apart.

Bake for 10 to 15 minutes the preheated oven, until golden.

Bold Vegan Chili

Ingredients

1 (12 ounce) package vegetarian burger crumbles
3 (15.25 ounce) cans kidney beans
1 large red onion, chopped
4 stalks celery, diced
2 red bell peppers, chopped
4 bay leaves
2 tablespoons hot chili powder
3 tablespoons molasses
1 cube vegetable bouillon
1 tablespoon chopped fresh cilantro
1 teaspoon hot pepper sauce
salt and pepper to taste
1 cup water
3 tablespoons all-purpose flour
1 cup hot water

Directions

In a slow cooker combine vegetarian crumbles, kidney beans, onion, celery, bell pepper, bay leaves, chili powder, molasses, bouillon, cilantro, hot sauce, salt, pepper and 1 cup water. Cook on high for 3 hours.

Dissolve flour in 1 cup hot water. Pour into chili and cook 1 more hour.

Vegan Hot and Sour Soup

Ingredients

1 ounce dried wood ear mushrooms
4 dried shiitake mushrooms
12 dried tiger lily buds
2 cups hot water
1/3 ounce bamboo fungus
3 tablespoons soy sauce
5 tablespoons rice vinegar
1/4 cup cornstarch
1 (8 ounce) container firm tofu, cut into 1/4 inch strips
1 quart vegetable broth
1/4 teaspoon crushed red pepper flakes
1/2 teaspoon ground black pepper
3/4 teaspoon ground white pepper
1/2 tablespoon chili oil
1/2 tablespoon sesame oil
1 green onion, sliced
1 cup Chinese dried mushrooms

Directions

In a small bowl, place wood mushrooms, shiitake mushrooms, and lily buds in 1 1/2 cups hot water. Soak 20 minutes, until rehydrated. Drain, reserving liquid. Trim stems from the mushrooms, and cut into thin strips. Cut the lily buds in half.

In a separate small bowl, soak bamboo fungus in 1/4 cup lightly salted hot water. Soak about 20 minutes, until rehydrated. Drain, and mince.

In a third small bowl, blend soy sauce, rice vinegar, and 1 tablespoon cornstarch. Place 1/2 the tofu strips into the mixture.

In a medium saucepan, mix the reserved mushroom and lily bud liquid with the vegetable broth. Bring to a boil, and stir in the wood mushrooms, shiitake mushrooms, and lily buds. Reduce heat, and simmer 3 to 5 minutes. Season with red pepper, black pepper, and white pepper.

In a small bowl, mix remaining cornstarch and remaining water. Stir into the broth mixture until thickened.

Mix soy sauce mixture and remaining tofu strips into the saucepan. Return to boil, and stir in the bamboo fungus, chili oil, and sesame oil. Garnish with green onion to serve.

Vegan Banana Blueberry Muffins

Ingredients

2 very ripe bananas, mashed
1/2 cup white sugar
1/2 teaspoon baking powder
1/2 teaspoon salt
3/4 cup all-purpose flour
1/2 cup whole wheat pastry flour
1 1/2 teaspoons egg replacer (dry)
2 tablespoons water
1/2 cup blueberries

Directions

Preheat oven to 350 degrees F (175 degrees C). Grease muffin cups or line with paper muffin liners.

In a large bowl combine mashed bananas, sugar, baking powder, salt and flours; mix until smooth. In a small bowl or cup combine egg replacer and water; stir into banana mixture. Fold in blueberries.

Spoon batter evenly, about 1/4 cup each, into muffin cups.

Bake in preheated oven for 20 to 25 minutes, or until golden brown.

Spicy Vegan Potato Curry

Ingredients

4 potatoes, peeled and cubed
2 tablespoons vegetable oil
1 yellow onion, diced
3 cloves garlic, minced
2 teaspoons ground cumin
1 1/2 teaspoons cayenne pepper
4 teaspoons curry powder
4 teaspoons garam masala
1 (1 inch) piece fresh ginger root, peeled and minced
2 teaspoons salt
1 (14.5 ounce) can diced tomatoes
1 (15 ounce) can garbanzo beans (chickpeas), rinsed and drained
1 (15 ounce) can peas, drained
1 (14 ounce) can coconut milk

Directions

Place potatoes into a large pot and cover with salted water. Bring to a boil over high heat, then reduce heat to medium-low, cover, and simmer until just tender, about 15 minutes. Drain and allow to steam dry for a minute or two.

Meanwhile, heat the vegetable oil in a large skillet over medium heat. Stir in the onion and garlic; cook and stir until the onion has softened and turned translucent, about 5 minutes. Season with cumin, cayenne pepper, curry powder, garam masala, ginger, and salt; cook for 2 minutes more. Add the tomatoes, garbanzo beans, peas, and potatoes. Pour in the coconut milk, and bring to a simmer. Simmer 5 to 10 minutes before serving.

Vegan Brownies

Ingredients

2 cups unbleached all-purpose flour
2 cups white sugar
3/4 cup unsweetened cocoa powder
1 teaspoon baking powder
1 teaspoon salt
1 cup water
1 cup vegetable oil
1 teaspoon vanilla extract

Directions

Preheat the oven to 350 degrees F (175 degrees C).

In a large bowl, stir together the flour, sugar, cocoa powder, baking powder and salt. Pour in water, vegetable oil and vanilla; mix until well blended. Spread evenly in a 9x13 inch baking pan.

Bake for 25 to 30 minutes in the preheated oven, until the top is no longer shiny. Let cool for at least 10 minutes before cutting into squares.

World's Best Vegan Pancakes

Ingredients

4 cups self-rising flour
1 tablespoon white sugar
1 tablespoon custard powder
2 cups soy milk

Directions

In a large bowl, stir together the flour, sugar and custard powder. Mix in the soy milk with a whisk so there are no lumps.

Heat a griddle over medium heat, and coat with nonstick cooking spray. Spoon batter onto the surface, and cook until bubbles begin to form on the surface. Flip with a spatula and cook on the other side until golden.

Vegan Corn Bread

Ingredients

1 cup all-purpose flour
1 cup cornmeal
1/4 cup turbinado sugar
1 tablespoon baking powder
1 teaspoon salt
1 cup sweetened, plain soy milk
1/3 cup vegetable oil
1/4 cup soft silken tofu

Directions

Preheat an oven to 400 degrees F (200 degrees C). Grease a 7 inch square baking pan. Whisk together the flour, cornmeal, sugar, baking powder, and salt in a mixing bowl; set aside.

Place the soy milk, oil, and tofu into a blender. Cover, and puree until smooth. Make a well in the center of the cornmeal mixture. Pour the pureed tofu into the well, then stir in the cornmeal mixture until just moistened. Pour the batter into the prepared baking pan.

Bake in the preheated oven until a toothpick inserted into the center comes out clean, 20 to 25 minutes. Cut into 9 pieces, and serve warm.

Quick Vegan Spaghetti Sauce

Ingredients

1 (29 ounce) can tomato sauce
1 (6 ounce) can sliced
mushrooms, drained
1/2 cup chopped celery
1/4 cup diced red onion
1/4 cup raisins
1/4 cup chopped walnuts
1 tomato, quartered
1 large orange, quartered
1 tablespoon minced garlic

Directions

In a large, heavy saucepan combine tomato sauce, mushrooms, celery, red onion, raisins, walnuts, tomato, orange and garlic. Cook on medium-high until vegetables are tender, about 30 minutes.

Vegan Corn Muffins

Ingredients

1 1/2 teaspoons egg replacer (dry)
2 tablespoons water
1 cup yellow cornmeal
1/2 cup all-purpose flour
2 teaspoons baking powder
2 tablespoons white sugar
2 tablespoons vegetable oil
1 cup water
1/2 teaspoon salt

Directions

Preheat oven to 450 degrees F (230 degrees C). Grease six muffin cups or line with paper muffin liners.

In a small bowl, beat together egg replacer and water. In a separate bowl, combine cornmeal, flour, baking powder, sugar and salt. Add egg mixture, oil and water; stir until smooth. Spoon batter into prepared muffin tins using approximately 1/2 cup for each muffin.

Bake in pre-heated oven for 10 to 15 minutes, until a toothpick inserted into the center of a muffin comes out clean.

Vegan Potatoes au Gratin

Ingredients

6 large potatoes, peeled and cubed
1 1/4 cups vegetable broth, divided
2 tablespoons all-purpose flour
1 teaspoon seasoning salt
1/2 teaspoon ground black pepper
1/4 teaspoon dry mustard
1/8 teaspoon nutmeg
2 cups soy milk
1 1/2 cups shredded Cheddar-flavored soy cheese, divided
1 cup soft bread crumbs
3 teaspoons paprika

Directions

Preheat oven to 350 degrees F (175 degrees C).

Bring a large pot of salted water to a boil. Add potatoes and cook until tender but still firm, about 15 minutes. Drain and place in a 9 x 13 inch baking dish.

Meanwhile, in a small saucepan over high heat, boil 2 tablespoons of broth. Reduce heat to low. Stir in flour, seasoning salt, pepper, mustard and nutmeg. Gradually add soy milk, stirring constantly until thickened. Stir in half of the soy cheese. Stir constantly until cheese is melted. Pour over potatoes.

In a small bowl combine the remaining broth and the bread crumbs. Spoon evenly over potatoes. Top with remaining soy cheese. Sprinkle with paprika.

Bake in preheated oven for 20 minutes.

Vegan Split Pea Soup II

Ingredients

1 tablespoon extra virgin olive oil
1 carrot, chopped
1 stalk celery, chopped
1 small onion, chopped
1 teaspoon curry powder
1 cup yellow split peas
4 cups water
1 teaspoon salt

Directions

Heat olive oil in a large saucepan. Sautee carrot, onion, celery and curry for about 5 minutes. Add the water, peas and salt. Simmer, stirring occasionally, for 45 to 50 minutes, or until very thick.

Vegan-Friendly Caramel Buttercream

Ingredients

1/2 cup vegan margarine
1 cup brown sugar, not packed
1/4 cup soy milk
1 teaspoon vanilla extract
1/2 cup shortening
5 cups confectioners' sugar

Directions

Stir the margarine and brown sugar together in a pan. Bring to a boil over medium-high heat, stirring constantly, and cook for 1 minute until dark brown. Remove from heat, and whisk in the soy milk and vanilla extract until smooth.

Beat the shortening together with 2 cups confectioners' sugar in a mixing bowl until well blended. Continue beating, and gradually add the brown sugar mixture, alternating with the remaining confectioners' sugar.

Vegan Bean Taco Filling

Ingredients

1 tablespoon olive oil
1 onion, diced
2 cloves garlic, minced
1 bell pepper, chopped
2 (14.5 ounce) cans black beans,
rinsed, drained, and mashed
2 tablespoons yellow cornmeal
1 1/2 tablespoons cumin
1 teaspoon paprika
1 teaspoon cayenne pepper
1 teaspoon chili powder
1 cup salsa

Directions

Heat olive oil in a medium skillet over medium heat. Stir in onion, garlic, and bell pepper; cook until tender. Stir in mashed beans. Add the cornmeal. Mix in cumin, paprika, cayenne, chili powder, and salsa. Cover, and cook 5 minutes.

Vegan Split Pea Soup I

Ingredients

1 tablespoon vegetable oil
1 onion, chopped
1 bay leaf
3 cloves garlic, minced
2 cups dried split peas
1/2 cup barley
1 1/2 teaspoons salt
7 1/2 cups water
3 carrots, chopped
3 stalks celery, chopped
3 potatoes, diced
1/2 cup chopped parsley
1/2 teaspoon dried basil
1/2 teaspoon dried thyme
1/2 teaspoon ground black pepper

Directions

In a large pot over medium high heat, saute the oil, onion, bay leaf and garlic for 5 minutes, or until onions are translucent. Add the peas, barley, salt and water. Bring to a boil and reduce heat to low. Simmer for 2 hours, stirring occasionally.

Add the carrots, celery, potatoes, parsley, basil, thyme and ground black pepper. Simmer for another hour, or until the peas and vegetables are tender.

Vegan Agave Cornbread Muffins

Ingredients

1/2 cup cornmeal
1/2 cup whole-wheat pastry flour
1/2 teaspoon baking soda
1/2 teaspoon salt
1/2 cup applesauce
1/2 cup soy milk
1/4 cup agave nectar
2 tablespoons canola oil

Directions

Preheat oven to 325 degrees F (165 degrees C). Lightly grease a muffin pan.

Combine the cornmeal, flour, baking soda, and salt in a large bowl; stir in the applesauce, soy milk, and agave nectar. Slowly add the oil while stirring. Pour the mixture into the muffin pan.

Bake in the preheated oven until a toothpick or small knife inserted in the crown of a muffin comes out clean, 15 to 20 minutes.

Vegan Cupcakes

Ingredients

1 tablespoon apple cider vinegar
1 1/2 cups almond milk
2 cups all-purpose flour
1 cup white sugar
2 teaspoons baking powder
1/2 teaspoon baking soda
1/2 teaspoon salt
1/2 cup coconut oil, warmed until liquid
1 1/4 teaspoons vanilla extract

Directions

Preheat oven to 350 degrees F (175 degrees C). Grease two 12 cup muffin pans or line with 18 paper baking cups.

Measure the apple cider vinegar into a 2 cup measuring cup. Fill with almond milk to make 1 1/2 cups. Let stand until curdled, about 5 minutes. In a large bowl, Whisk together the flour, sugar, baking powder, baking soda and salt. In a separate bowl, whisk together the almond milk mixture, coconut oil and vanilla. Pour the wet ingredients into the dry ingredients and stir just until blended. Spoon the batter into the prepared cups, dividing evenly.

Bake in the preheated oven until the tops spring back when lightly pressed, 15 to 20 minutes. Cool in the pan set over a wire rack. When cool, arrange the cupcakes on a serving platter. Frost with desired frosting.

Spicy Thai Vegan Burger

Ingredients

1 cup fresh pea pods
1/2 cup shredded carrots
1/2 cup quartered cherry tomatoes
1/3 cup sliced green onions
2 tablespoons slivered fresh Thai basil or fresh basil
1/4 cup unsweetened light coconut milk or unsweetened coconut milk*
1 tablespoon lime juice
1/2 teaspoon toasted sesame oil or sesame seeds, toasted
1/4 teaspoon crushed red pepper
4 Morningstar FarmsB® GrillersB® Vegan Veggie Burgers
1 (9-inch) focaccia, cut into fourths and horizontally split

Directions

Lengthwise cut pea pods into slivers. In medium bowl toss together pea pods, carrots, tomatoes, green onions and basil. Set aside. In small bowl whisk together coconut milk, lime juice, sesame oil and red pepper. Drizzle over vegetables. Toss to coat.

Cook vegan veggie burgers according to package directions. Serve hot burgers in focaccia, topped with vegetable mixture.

ON THE GRILL: Preheat grill. Use a food thermometer to be sure patties reach minimum internal temperature of 160 degrees F.

Vegan Fajitas

Ingredients

1/4 cup olive oil
1/4 cup red wine vinegar
1 teaspoon dried oregano
1 teaspoon chili powder
garlic salt to taste
salt and pepper to taste
1 teaspoon white sugar

2 small zucchini, julienned
2 medium small yellow squash, julienned
1 large onion, sliced
1 green bell pepper, cut into thin strips
1 red bell pepper, cut into thin strips
2 tablespoons olive oil
1 (8.75 ounce) can whole kernel corn, drained
1 (15 ounce) can black beans, drained

Directions

In a large bowl combine olive oil, vinegar, oregano, chili powder, garlic salt, salt, pepper and sugar. To the marinade add the zucchini, yellow squash, onion, green pepper and red pepper. Marinate vegetables in the refrigerator for at least 30 minutes, but not more than 24 hours.

Heat oil in a large skillet over medium-high heat. Drain the vegetables and saute until tender, about 10 to 15 minutes. Stir in the corn and beans; increase the heat to high for 5 minutes, to brown vegetables.

Vegan Gelatin

Ingredients

1/2 teaspoon cornstarch
1 teaspoon water
2 cups cherry juice
1 teaspoon agar-agar

Directions

Dissolve the cornstarch in the water in a small cup or bowl and set aside. In a saucepan, combine 1 1/2 cups of cherry juice and agar-agar powder. Let stand for 5 minutes to soften. Set heat to medium-high and bring to a simmer. Simmer for 1 minute.

Remove from the heat and stir in the remaining juice along with the cornstarch mixture until no longer cloudy. Pour into small serving cups and refrigerate for 4 hours before serving.

Vegan Cheesecake

Ingredients

1 (12 ounce) package soft tofu
1/2 cup soy milk
1/2 cup white sugar
1 tablespoon vanilla extract
1/4 cup maple syrup
1 (9 inch) prepared graham cracker crust

Directions

Preheat oven to 350 degrees F (175 degrees C).

In a blender, combine the tofu, soy milk, sugar, vanilla extract and maple syrup. Blend until smooth and pour into pie crust.

Bake at 350 degrees F (175 degrees C) for 30 minutes. Remove from oven and allow to cool; refrigerate until chilled.

Vegan Borscht

Ingredients

1 tablespoon olive oil
3 cloves garlic, minced
1 onion, chopped
3 tablespoons olive oil
2 stalks celery, chopped (optional)
2 carrots, finely chopped
1 green bell pepper, chopped
3 beets, including greens, diced
1 (16 ounce) can whole peeled tomatoes
1/2 cup canned peeled and diced tomatoes
2 potatoes, quartered
1 cup shredded Swiss chard
2 cups vegetable broth
4 cups water
2 tablespoons dried dill weed
salt and freshly ground black pepper to taste
1 (16 ounce) package silken tofu

Directions

Heat 1 tablespoon of olive oil in a skillet over medium heat. Stir in the garlic and onion; cook and stir until the onion has softened and turned translucent, about 5 minutes. Set aside. Heat the remaining 3 tablespoons of olive oil in a large pot over medium-high heat. Stir in the celery, carrots, bell pepper, beets including the greens, whole tomatoes, diced tomatoes, potatoes, Swiss chard, and the onion mixture. Cook and stir until the chard begins to wilt, 4 to 8 minutes. Stir in the vegetable broth, water, dill weed, and salt and pepper. Bring to a boil, and reduce heat to low. Simmer for 1 hour.

Strain half the beets from the broth and place in a blender, filling the pitcher no more than halfway full. Hold down the lid of the blender with a folded kitchen towel, and carefully start the blender, using a few quick pulses to get the beets moving before leaving it on to puree. Add the tofu, and continue pureeing until smooth. Stir the tofu mixture back into the pot. Simmer until the mixture is reduced by a third, about another hour. Serve chilled or warm.

Vegan Yogurt Sundae

Ingredients

1/4 cup frozen berries
1 tablespoon white sugar
2 tablespoons vegan chocolate chips
1 tablespoon vegan margarine
3 tablespoons soy milk or soy creamer
1 (8 ounce) container vanilla soy yogurt
1 tablespoon chopped nuts

Directions

Toss berries with sugar in a microwave safe bowl. Cook in the microwave for 40 seconds at full power until thawed.

Place chocolate chips and margarine in a microwave safe bowl. Cook in the microwave at 60% power for 45 seconds until melted. Use a fork to stir until smooth, then stir in soy milk until incorporated; set aside.

Spoon the soy yogurt into a small bowl, then spoon fruit overtop. Pour on chocolate sauce and sprinkle with nuts.

Vegan Pumpkin Ice Cream

Ingredients

1/4 cup soy creamer
2 tablespoons arrowroot powder
1 3/4 cups soy creamer
1 cup soy milk
3/4 cup brown sugar
1 cup pumpkin puree
1 teaspoon vanilla extract
1 1/2 teaspoons pumpkin pie spice

Directions

Mix 1/4 cup soy creamer with arrowroot and set aside. Whisk together 1 3/4 cup soy creamer, soy milk, brown sugar, pumpkin puree, vanilla extract, and pumpkin pie spice in a saucepan over medium heat, stirring frequently, until just boiling. Remove the pan from the heat; stir in the arrowroot mixture to thicken. Set aside to cool for 30 minutes.

Fill cylinder of ice cream freezer; freeze according to manufacturer's directions.

Vegan Chunky Chili

Ingredients

1/2 cup dry kidney beans, soaked overnight
1/2 cup dry white beans, soaked overnight
1/2 cup dry brown lentils, soaked overnight
6 cups chopped fresh tomatoes
6 cups water
1 cup chopped fresh mushrooms
1/2 cup chopped green bell pepper
1/2 cup chopped red bell pepper
1/2 cup fresh green beans
1/2 cup chopped celery
1/4 onion, chopped
1/4 red onion, chopped
3/4 cup extra firm tofu, drained, crumbled
salt to taste
black pepper to taste
onion powder to taste
garlic powder to taste
chili powder to taste

Directions

Drain and rinse kidney beans, white beans and lentils. Combine in a large pot and cover with water; boil over medium-high to high heat for 1 hour, or until tender.

Meanwhile, in a large saucepan over high heat, combine tomatoes and water; bring to a boil. Reduce heat to low and simmer, uncovered, for 1 hour, or until tomatoes are broken down.

Stir the tomatoes into the beans and add mushrooms, green bell pepper, red bell pepper, green beans, celery, onions and tofu. Season with salt, pepper, onion powder, garlic powder and chili powder to taste. Simmer for 2 to 3 hours, or until desired consistency is reached.

Vegan Lasagna II

Ingredients

3 cloves garlic, minced
1/2 pound mushrooms
1 tablespoon vegetable oil
1 (10.75 ounce) can tomato puree
1 (10 ounce) package frozen spinach, thawed and drained
2 teaspoons garlic salt
2 tablespoons Italian-style seasoning
1 (12 ounce) package soft tofu
2/3 (16 ounce) package instant lasagna noodles

Directions

Preheat oven to 375 degrees F (190 degrees C).

In a large skillet, saute garlic and mushrooms in oil until all the liquid is cooked out. Add 1/3 tomato puree to mushrooms and garlic, cook 2 to 3 minutes, and remove from heat.

In a microwave-safe bowl, combine spinach, garlic salt, Italian seasoning and tofu. Blend until the mixture is an even consistency. Heat in a microwave on high for 2 minutes.

In a 9x9 inch baking pan, pour one thin layer of remaining tomato puree, a layer of noodles, 1/2 the tofu mixture, the mushroom sauce, a layer of noodles, 1/2 the tofu mixture, a layer of tomato puree, a layer of noodles, and a final layer of tomato puree.

Bake 45 minutes in the preheated oven.

Vegan Carrot Cake

Ingredients

2 cups whole wheat flour
1/4 cup soy flour (optional)
1 1/2 tablespoons ground cinnamon
1 tablespoon ground cloves
4 teaspoons baking soda
2 teaspoons tapioca starch (optional)
1/2 teaspoon salt
1 1/2 cups hot water
1/4 cup flax seed meal
2 cups packed brown sugar
4 teaspoons vanilla extract
3/4 cup dried currants (optional)
6 carrots, grated
1/2 cup blanched slivered almonds (optional)

Directions

Preheat oven to 350 degrees F (175 degrees C). Prepare a 9x13 inch baking pan with cooking spray. Whisk together the whole wheat flour, soy flour, cinnamon, ground cloves, baking soda, tapioca starch, and salt in a bowl until blended; set aside.

Pour the hot water into a mixing bowl, and sprinkle with the flax meal. Stir for a minute until the flax begins to absorb the water, and the mixture slightly thickens. Stir in the brown sugar and vanilla until the sugar has dissolved, then add the currants, carrots, and almonds. Stir in the dry mixture until just moistened, then pour into the prepared pan.

Bake in the preheated oven until a toothpick inserted into the center comes out clean, about 30 minutes. Cool in the pan for 10 minutes before removing to cool completely on a wire rack.

Vegan Mexican Stew

Ingredients

5 medium potatoes, peeled and cubed
2 carrots, chopped
1 stalk celery, chopped
4 1/2 cups water
4 cubes vegetable bouillon
1 tablespoon olive oil
1 large onion, diced
4 cloves garlic, minced
1 tablespoon chili powder
1 tablespoon cumin
1 1/2 tablespoons seasoned salt
1 (29 ounce) can hominy, drained
1 (28 ounce) can diced tomatoes with green chile peppers
salt and pepper to taste

Directions

Place the potatoes, carrots, and celery in a pot with enough lightly salted water to cover, and bring to a boil. Cook about 10 minutes, until slightly tender. Drain, and set aside.

Place the 4 1/2 cups water and vegetable bouillon cubes in a pot. Bring to a boil, and cook until bouillon cubes have dissolved. Remove from heat, and set aside.

Heat the olive oil in a large pot. Saute the onion and garlic until tender. Season with chili powder, cumin, and seasoned salt. Mix in the potatoes, carrots, and celery. Cook and stir about 2 minutes, until heated through. Mix in the water and dissolved bouillon cube mixture, hominy, and diced tomatoes with green chiles. Bring to a boil, reduce heat, and simmer 45 minutes. Season with salt and pepper to taste.

Tangy Vegan Crockpot Corn Chowder

Ingredients

2 (12 ounce) cans whole kernel corn
3 cups vegetable broth
3 potatoes, diced
1 large onion, diced
1 clove garlic, minced
2 red chile peppers, minced
1 tablespoon chili powder
2 teaspoons salt
1 tablespoon parsley flakes
black pepper to taste
1 3/4 cups soy milk
1/4 cup margarine
1 lime, juiced

Directions

Place the corn, vegetable broth, potatoes, onion, garlic, red chile peppers, chili powder, salt, parsley, and black pepper in a slow cooker; cover. Cook on Low for 7 hours.

Pour the vegetable mixture into a blender, filling the pitcher no more than halfway full. Hold the lid of the blender with a folded kitchen towel and carefully start the blender using a few quick pulses before leaving it on to puree. Puree in batches until smooth and pour into a clean pot. Alternately, you can use a stick blender and puree the mixture in the cooking pot. Once everything has been pureed, return it to the slow cooker. Stir the soy milk and margarine to the mixture; cook on Low for 1 hour more. Add the lime juice to serve.

Traditional Style Vegan Shepherd's Pie

Ingredients

Mashed potato layer:
5 russet potatoes, peeled and cut into 1-inch cubes
1/2 cup vegan mayonnaise
1/2 cup soy milk
1/4 cup olive oil
3 tablespoons vegan cream cheese substitute (such as Tofutti ®)
2 teaspoons salt

Bottom layer:
1 tablespoon vegetable oil
1 large yellow onion, chopped
2 carrots, chopped
3 stalks celery, chopped
1/2 cup frozen peas
1 tomato, chopped
1 teaspoon Italian seasoning
1 clove garlic, minced, or more to taste
1 pinch ground black pepper to taste
1 (14 ounce) package vegetarian ground beef substitute

1/2 cup shredded Cheddar-style soy cheese

Directions

Place the potatoes in a pot, cover with cold water, and bring to a boil over medium-high heat. Turn the heat to medium-low, and boil the potatoes until tender, about 25 minutes; drain.

Stir the vegan mayonnaise, soy milk, olive oil, vegan cream cheese, and salt into the potatoes, and mash with a potato masher until smooth and fluffy. Set the potatoes aside.

Preheat oven to 400 degrees F (200 degrees C), and spray a 2-quart baking dish with cooking spray.

Heat the vegetable oil in a large skillet over medium heat, and cook and stir the onion, carrots, celery, frozen peas, and tomato until softened, about 10 minutes. Stir in the Italian seasoning, garlic, and pepper.

Reduce the heat to medium-low, and crumble the vegetarian ground beef substitute into the skillet with the vegetables. Cook and stir, breaking up the meat substitute, until the mixture is hot, about 5 minutes.

Spread the vegetarian meat substitute mixture into the bottom of the baking dish, and top with the mashed potatoes, smoothing them into an even layer. Sprinkle the potatoes with the shredded soy cheese.

Bake in the preheated oven until the cheese is melted and slightly browned and the casserole is hot, about 20 minutes.

Yummy Vegan Pesto Classico

Ingredients

1/3 cup pine nuts
2/3 cup olive oil
5 cloves garlic
1/3 cup nutritional yeast
1 bunch fresh basil leaves
salt and pepper to taste

Directions

Place the pine nuts in a skillet over medium heat, and cook, stirring constantly, until lightly toasted.

Gradually mix the pine nuts, olive oil, garlic, nutritional yeast, and basil in a food processor, and process until smooth. Season with salt and pepper.

Vegan Baked Beans

Ingredients

1 (16 ounce) package dry navy beans
6 cups water
2 tablespoons olive oil
2 cups chopped sweet onions
1 clove garlic, minced
4 (8 ounce) cans tomato sauce
1/4 cup firmly packed brown sugar
1/4 cup molasses
2 tablespoons cider vinegar
3 bay leaves
1 teaspoon dry mustard
1/4 teaspoon ground black pepper
1/4 teaspoon ground nutmeg
1/4 teaspoon ground cinnamon

Directions

Place beans and water in a large pot, and bring to a boil. Reduce heat to medium, and continue cooking 1 hour, stirring occasionally, until beans are tender. Drain, and transfer to a large casserole dish.

Preheat oven to 300 degrees F (150 degrees C).

Heat the olive oil in a skillet over medium heat. Stir in the onions, and cook until tender. Mix in garlic, and cook until golden brown. Mix onions and garlic into casserole dish with the beans. Stir in the tomato sauce. Mix in brown sugar, molasses, vinegar, bay leaves, mustard, pepper, nutmeg, and cinnamon.

Cover and bake 3 1/2 hours in the preheated oven, stirring frequently and adding water if necessary. Remove cover, and continue baking 30 minutes.

Delicious Vegan Hot Chocolate

Ingredients

2 1/2 cups soy milk
3 tablespoons white sugar
3 tablespoons cocoa powder
1/2 teaspoon salt
1/2 teaspoon vanilla extract
1 pinch ground cinnamon
1 pinch cayenne pepper

Directions

Bring the soy milk, sugar, cocoa powder, salt, vanilla extract, cinnamon, and cayenne pepper to a simmer in a saucepan over medium-high heat. Remove from the heat and whisk until frothy. Serve immediately.

Vegan Cream 'Cheese' Frosting

Ingredients

1/2 cup vegan cream cheese substitute (such as Tofutti®„ӳ)
1/2 cup soy margarine
1 teaspoon vanilla extract
1/4 cup soy flour
2 cups confectioners' sugar

Directions

Beat the cream cheese and margarine together with the vanilla extract in a mixing bowl with an electric hand mixer until light. Beat in the soy flour, followed by the confectioners' sugar until light and fluffy. Refrigerate at least 20 minutes before using.

Easy Vegan Pasta Sauce

Ingredients

1 teaspoon vegetable oil
1/2 small yellow onion, diced
2 cloves garlic, minced
5 large tomatoes, cubed
1 small green bell pepper, diced
1/2 teaspoon salt
1/2 teaspoon black pepper
1 teaspoon dried basil leaves
1/2 teaspoon dried oregano

Directions

In a skillet over medium-low heat, saute onion and garlic in the vegetable oil. Place tomatoes into onion and garlic mixture. Stir in diced bell pepper, salt, pepper, basil and oregano. Let simmer for 20 minutes, stirring occasionally. Turn down heat if it starts to stick.

Vegan Goddess Dressing

Ingredients

1 (10 ounce) package soft silken tofu
1/3 cup olive oil
1/4 cup chopped fresh basil
1/2 teaspoon rice vinegar
1/4 teaspoon salt
3 teaspoons tamari

Directions

Whisk together the tofu and olive oil until a thick mayonnaise like consistency is reached.

Add the herbs, vinegar, salt and soy sauce; mix well and refrigerate.

Vegan Mac and No Cheese

Ingredients

1 (8 ounce) package uncooked elbow macaroni
1 tablespoon vegetable oil
1 medium onion, chopped
1 cup cashews
1/3 cup lemon juice
1 1/3 cups water
salt to taste
1/3 cup canola oil
4 ounces roasted red peppers, drained
3 tablespoons nutritional yeast
1 teaspoon garlic powder
1 teaspoon onion powder

Directions

Preheat oven to 350 degrees F (175 degrees C).

Bring a large pot of lightly salted water to a boil. Add macaroni, and cook for 8 to 10 minutes or until al dente; drain. Transfer to a medium baking dish.

Heat vegetable oil in a medium saucepan over medium heat. Stir in onion, and cook until tender and lightly browned. Gently mix with the macaroni.

In a blender or food processor, mix cashews, lemon juice, water, and salt. Gradually blend in canola oil, roasted red peppers, nutritional yeast, garlic powder, and onion powder. Blend until smooth. Thoroughly mix with the macaroni and onions.

Bake 45 minutes in the preheated oven, until lightly browned. Cool 10 to 15 minutes before serving.

Vegan Pumpkin Nog

Ingredients

1 (29 ounce) can pumpkin puree
4 cups vanilla rice milk
1 cup vanilla flavored non-dairy frozen dessert
1 teaspoon ground cinnamon
1/4 teaspoon ground nutmeg
1/4 teaspoon ground mace

Directions

Combine the pumpkin, rice milk, rice milk ice cream, cinnamon, nutmeg and mace in a blender. Puree until smooth. Add additional rice milk to thin, if desired.

Vegan Chili

Ingredients

1 (12 ounce) package vegetarian burger crumbles
1 (15 ounce) can tomato sauce
1 cup water
1 small onion, chopped
3 cloves garlic, minced
1 tablespoon vegetarian Worcestershire sauce
1 teaspoon liquid smoke flavoring
2 teaspoons chili powder
1/8 teaspoon black pepper
1 teaspoon dry mustard
1 teaspoon salt
1/8 teaspoon red pepper flakes

Directions

In a large pot combine crumbles, tomato sauce, water, onion, garlic, Worcestershire sauce, liquid smoke, chili powder, black pepper, mustard, salt and pepper flakes. Cook on low heat for 30 minutes, or until heated through.

Vegan Sun-Dried Tomato Pesto

Ingredients

2 cups fresh basil leaves
5 sun-dried tomatoes, softened
3 cloves garlic, crushed 1/4 teaspoon salt
3 tablespoons toasted pine nuts 1/4 cup olive oil

Directions

Place basil, tomatoes, garlic, salt, and nuts in an electric food processor or blender.
Puree. Add olive oil slowly, and blend slowly until the mixture is to your desired texture.

Vegan Sun-Dried Tomato Pesto

Vegetarian Diet Cookbook 2021

The Beginner's Guide to Discover The Health Benefits of Eating a Plant Based Diet: Over 90 Quick, Easy, Inspired and Flexible Recipes for Eating Well Without Meat

Richard Tillcot

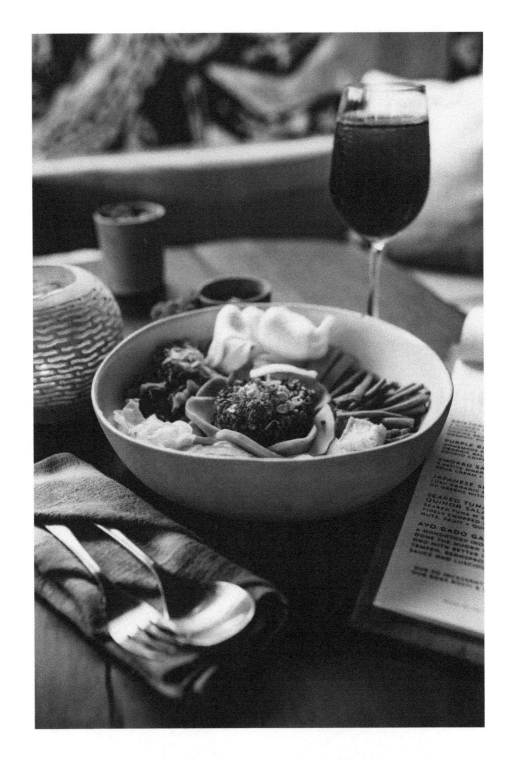

LET'S START!

INTRODUCTION

It's always hard to accept and undergo changes; likewise altering to a vegetarian diet is not as easy as it may be presumed.

So, it is very important to do an in-depth analysis before adapting to a new lifestyle. Sometimes, switching over to meatless diet might be difficult.

Therefore, it is better to know the positive and negative effects beforehand, because becoming vegetarian involves a lot more than just cutting on meat.

There are several types of vegetarians like some who prefer eating fish and whereas some who don't. On the other hand, there are people who even do not consume dairy products including cheese and eggs, and live on fruits and vegetables.

Switching to a vegetarian diet is always an individual's preference. One must also keep in mind the nutritional supplements that body would require, before you shun cottage cheese and other nutritional foods that provide essential nourishment.

It is better to start off slowly and progress gradually to be a total vegetarian. Though it is hard to believe, the entire body system will go through definite changes, since the body will not be getting something which it is very much habitual of.

It is always better to reduce the quantity gradually, instead depriving meat from the routine diet suddenly, replace it by in-taking fish or chicken and then start cutting down the consumption gradually turning to be a total vegetarian.

The most important part in turning to a vegetarian style is to know the nutritional contents in the food which would be consumed instead of meat. Generally, those who do not approve of a vegetarian lifestyle, have an assumption that their body would be deprived of vital vitamins and minerals, if meat is not added in the diet.

Although, there are many who have been successful in switching over to a meatless diet. Such individuals have been able to supply their body with necessary nutrients and hence filling in the lag caused by the meatless diet.

Many researches have proved that green vegetables like broccoli, kale and spinach contains enormous amounts of calcium and consumption of these green vegetables would give necessary nutrients to stay healthy.

As well, nuts are known to be rich source of protein. Consumption of such vegetarian diets can ensure that one gets enough to have a healthy life with balanced nutrition.

Turning to a vegetarian diet is one of the vital aspects that you can do to make your body feel healthy. And for individuals already converted to a vegan style, must have realized that they feel great and have excessive energy and also were able lose weight without starving. So, start thinking on this and make a progress towards a satisfying lifestyle.

HOW TO BECOME A VEGETARIAN

It may possibly seem impractical to imagine the initiatives a person should take to study to turn to a vegetarian diet.

Nevertheless, it is not as simple as merely hacking meat out of one's diet? The response to that straightforward issue is.... not actually. People perceive that becoming a vegan requires much more effort, than simply refusing to a steak or a hamburger.

An individual would discover that exploring to become a vegan entails a lot of examination and also some serious efforts, so that one can be fit and not devoid their body of something that it essentially requires to function completely in the manner it was intended to.

The most important thing one requires to attempt when turning to a vegan diet is to take it leisurely. If you have been habitual of consuming meat for years now, in that case a laid-back attitude will not make much difference. You will have to make some serious and planned efforts to become a vegan. Begin by slashing meat out of your regular diet gradually.

You can cut on meat for some days and then switch over to consuming fish or chicken. This process can eventually help you in quitting meat permanently as the body slowly and progressively gets used change in diet.

If an individual desire to realize how to adopt a lacta-vegetarian diet, then they will also have to do petite exploration into the nutrients that are comprised in different vegetables, so a person can be certain that their body is receiving the essential stuff it requires to be well-built as well as efficient. It must be kept in mind that vitamins like B and C as well as minerals like iron and zinc are essential for the human.

Calcium and protein are also vital components of a proportionate diet, so one would wish to know the nutritional value of the food that they are consuming. It is necessary to ensure that the body is provided all the essential nutrients and vitamins that it requires to function efficiently.

For the reason that people are removing meat from their diet, they must ensure that they intake sufficient protein into their body. Protein is crucial for the human body and hence when people are studying how to turn into a vegan, they will desire to get substitute supplies of protein in order that their body can work the manner it was intended to.

Eating Healthy Vegetarian

Vegan diets are known to be very hale and hearty, but eating a reasonable food when an individual is a vegetarian, it usually attracts little additional notice. When a person shuns red meat and animal protein out of their diet, they are shunning out a chief resource of protein which their body requires. It means that eating healthy diet as a vegan will entail adding foods into one's diet that will endow with nutrients commonly found in meat foodstuffs.

By exploring a diet consisting of fruits, vegetables, and whole grains, people can easily avail the vitamins and nutrients they want from vegetarian sources so that their vegetarian way of life is healthy and in proportion.

By consuming food items like legumes, soy foods, nuts, and eggs, one can obtain the essential protein content that they require to nurture. One must also keep in mind that other nutrients like the minerals iron, calcium and the vitamins D and B12, are equally vital for vegans.

Whereas it's factual that removing meat out of one's diet and consuming a diet rich in vegetables, fruits, and grains is healthy. But vegetarians require worrying about other things essential nutrients like receiving the right balance of vitamins and minerals from their diet.

Many can constantly take a vitamin add-on, but since a lot of these supplements include animal derivatives, many devoted vegetarians hesitate in taking them. It is essential that one must look out for a diet which is rich in vitamins B and C, iron and niacin since they are also vital part of a healthy lacto-vegetarian way of life.

A person doesn't have to forgo one's health when they prefer to become a vegan. Ingestion of healthy vegetarian diet is not an easy task. One must exclusively take leisure time to study and find food items that include nutrients most essential for the body. For this, perhaps you will have to go extensively through several books, magazines or even surf internet.

People can make all kinds of swaps in their diet that can replace meat when aren't eating any longer. For instance, one can opt for soy milk as an alternative to cow's milk which in turn will provide the necessary calcium to the body. Including nuts and grains into a vegetarian diet suitably turns it into a healthy diet. Also, nuts and grains are full of proteins which are helpful in developing healthy bones.

Several Studies have revealed that vegetarians generally have healthy eating routine that leads to a fit and healthy body. They also have a higher tendency to remain healthy and energetic. The thing people need to keep in mind for healthy vegan diet is that they have to give particular interest to the nutrient content present in the foods that they eat and be sure to eat balanced diet.

VEGETARIAN WEIGHT LOSS DIET

Many people choose to become vegetarians because they need to go on a weight loss diet but hate the idea of starving themselves.

A vegetarian diet can aid in weight loss in many, many ways because you are cutting out all red meat which can contain a lot of fat that is stored in your body's cells and really packs on the pounds. A vegetarian eats a lot of fruits and vegetables as well as fish and seafood which is all healthy for you and can be a great weight loss tool.

Going on a diet is difficult because you want to achieve your weight loss goal which is why you will really want to consider a vegetarian lifestyle change.

Vegetables are naturally low in calories and good for you, so you won't have to worry about packing on the pounds with them.

Fruits, while they are good for you, contain a lot of water and can make you weigh more since the body tends to retain water, but know that you are still eating healthy.

A good, well-balance vegetarian diet made for maximum weight loss contains a variety of foods and spices that taste good and make you feel full. You see, foods become fattening because of how we prepare them and what we add to them.

You can have a bowl full of healthy mushrooms, but if you cook them in butter and add in some heavy cream to make a soup, you have packed on the calories and negated the naturally healthy effects.

When you are on a vegetarian diet for weight loss, stay away from frying your foods to the extent that you possibly can. If you want to sauté some of your veggies, do so in an extra virgin olive oil (or EVOO as Rachel Ray says) which is lower in caloric content and provides some of the good fats that your body needs.

You will also want to stay away from high-fat cheeses and opt for the lower- fat varieties and explore substitutions such as using plain yogurt for sour cream.

A vegetarian diet is a great weight loss tool as well a healthy way to eat. Once you have achieved your weight loss goals, we're willing to bet that you will continue with your vegetarian diet.

Going meatless isn't as difficult as many people think it is. You will find yourself with more energy, quicker metabolism (which burns fat), and a smaller grocery bill - especially if you grow most of your vegetables.

So, for maximum weight loss, opt for the vegetarian diet and watch the pounds melt off without feeling hungry all the time.

BEING A VEGETARIAN

Being vegetarian is a great way to health. It not only helps in retrieval of in-store metabolism but eventually leads to a much healthier lifestyle.

Often, we see people around us who have to adopt a proper diet due to some disease that they might have caught up due to improper diet. Since meat eaters are more prone to cholesterol deposition and diabetes, being vegetarian, it could help them keeping a proper check of their health.

When we are considering vegetarians in general view such people would be imagined as eating a lot of green salad, but this view is slightly misconceived, as on a wider perspective the classification is much different than considered.

Below are the few mentioned classifications:

• Lacto-ovo-vegetarian- People who prefer eating both the dairy products and eggs. This is the most commonly preferred diet by vegetarians.

• Lacto-vegetarians-Under this category people consume dairy products but they do not consume egg.

• Vegan-People who do not consume any of the dairy products, eggs or any of the animal products.

• Fruitarian-Categorized under vegan is such a classification in which consumption of processed food is minimized up to optimum level. It comprises of mainly raw fruits, grain and nuts. Since fruitarians believe in consumption of only that food which could be harvested only without killing the plant.

• Macrobiotic-This type of diet is followed for spiritual and philosophical reasons. It is taken in consideration with a perspective of negative and positive energies that food contains. The yin is the positive attribute while the yang being its negative attribute.

This style of eating aims at maintaining a proper diet. As this diet advances through ten levels, it gets narrowed down.

All of the level does comprise vegetarians but eventually eliminates animal product and in extreme cases eliminating even fruits and vegetables leading to a diet that consists of only brown rice.

Everyone have their own reasons so as to why they have chosen to be a vegetarian like some chose to be vegetarians just because they do not want to be cruel to animals while others prefer it just considering it being a much healthier choice. Reason could be any but it has been medically proven as well that vegetarian people lead a much greater deal of healthy life.

Vegetarians are less prone to cholesterol deposition, diabetes and even eliminating risks of some forms of cancer as well. Organic food is grown with minimized use of pesticides hence removing the risk of harmful chemicals being consumed, about which the scientists have proven to cause serious damage to the proper functioning of the body and nervous system.

If this in some way has persuaded you to choose a vegetarian life style then go ahead and step towards a much healthier life. Initially it could be very demanding and difficult but in long run it would bring about drastic changes leading to a much safer and better health.

VEGETARIAN SPORTS NUTRITION

Let's say you are highly involved in sports, but you are a vegan and are worried about getting the right nutrition.

Don't worry. You can get all the nutrition you need while still living your vegetarian lifestyle and participating in sports. You are not required to make sacrifices in your diet just because you don't want to eat meat.

In fact, you might actually find that a vegetarian diet is extremely conducive to allowing you to participate in sports because the nutrition you will find in vegetables, fruits, and grains will actually give you more energy.

The first thing you need to remember is that you must eat before a workout so that your body can begin to process the food and give you the nutritional requirements you need to sustain a heavy work out and be able to have enough energy to participate in the sports that you like to do.

That means that vegetarians must get a lot of carbohydrates before they play sports and then let the nutrition that is contained in those carb loaded foods work for you.

You will also need to eat a good vegetarian meal after you are done participating in sports so that you can replenish the nutrition that is naturally lost through sweat during your workout.

However, you will want to avoid carbs as much as possible in this meal since carbs can easily be converted into fat and actually negate all of the benefits you have just given yourself.

If you are heavily involved in sports and you are a lacto-vegetarian, we recommend that you get a large number of nuts and grains which are filled with carbohydrates as well as a lot of fruits that can give your body some highly needed water that will eventually be sweated out during your sports workout.

Athletes who are vegetarians often worry about their nutrition since participating in sports is so important to keeping them fit. All they really need to remember is that the body needs certain vitamins and minerals to function correctly. That's where research comes into play.

Ask some of your vegetarian friends what they do before they play sports so that their nutrition doesn't suffer. Look online for suggestions about what you can do to get the most nutrition from your vegetarian diet before playing sports.

Read books and ask your doctor along the way if you are worried about nutrition as a vegetarian who participates heavily in sports. The old saying is that you can never have too much information, so seek out what is there for you and then take heed. It will all be worth it in the end!

LOW CARB VEGETARIAN

Human bodies need various nutrients to stay fit. Being vegetarian is good, but you need to balance the vitamins and nutrients skillfully. The only thing that should come in your mind is the balance of carbs.

Carbs are a great source of energy and that is the only reason to consume carbs in proper proportion. Excess of carbs in a vegetarian diet will trigger fat production in human body. Carbs alter sugar which in turn changes into fat and this creates problem if the quantity of conversion is in excess.

Some foods are rich in carbohydrates like rice, potato and grains, so if you have plans to low down on carb intake, you should minimize the consumption of such foods. It is also not advisable to completely cut these foods in your diet as these are good source of carbs. Efforts should be done to curtail the consumption of these food products.

Carbs are also present in flour which also includes the whole wheat flour. You should avoid or minimize eating bread, if you are serious about the proper carbs intake. Make sure, that the source of your carbs is appropriate to control the suitable consumption of carbs. Stay away from white bread and eat whole grain bread to compensate the carb requirement of body.

Being vegetarian is good, but you have to give up lot of things during the process. The diet should include a lot of fresh and green vegetables.

Selection of oils for preparing the food should also be taken into account. If you are using olive oil you must use the proper quantity to reach the required level of carb. Also consider steaming and grilling of oil in order to ensure low carb intake. You have the natural vitamins in green and leafy vegetables.

Don't consume carbohydrates that will make you gain weight.

Different people have different reasons for changing their lifestyle to a vegetarian one. The most basic reason is losing extra weight. Some people also are really concerned about killing of various animals. A well-balanced diet is the most important criteria behind a vegetarian lifestyle. Excess amount of carbohydrates can change into sugar which can gradually lead to gaining extra weight.

Before you follow a vegetarian diet that is also low in carbohydrate content, you must be very careful in finding the exact amount of carbohydrate present in your diet. If the amount of carbs is very low, then it may affect your body and most importantly your health. The most important part of a healthy diet is nutrition.

Low Calorie Vegetarian Recipes

Maybe an individual would have preferred a vegetarian standard of living for the reason that they wish to drop weight and require low calorie vegan approach to aid them in their weight loss objectives. The excellent news is that merely by changing over to meat free eating; one would be ingesting low calories. The unrevealed aspect of preparing healthy vegan recipes is to remove the additional flab that makes meals filling.

Initially, when a person is preparing low-fat vegan recipes, people will want to avoid the use of too much oil. An individual can, yet use a superior quality additional virgin olive oil for tastings and salads. EVOO has less caloric value and gives some of the "beneficial fats" that our body need.

Discourage fried foods while you are preparing vegetarian recipes which are less in caloric value.

Even if one does use the added virgin olive oil for frying, in spite of this, fried foods characteristically have higher calories, so one should shun fried foods as much as feasible.

Steam the vegetables as an alternative and refrain from boiling them. Boiling will deplete the significant nutrients. Grill vegetables for some change. You can also apply a no calorie or light cooking spray to provide them some wetness or even scatter on a little watery lemon juice.

If one's diet permits them to eat seafood, boil fish in spite of frying it. It is advisable to grill the fish since grilling is an immense mode to add taste and distinctiveness to their foods. Spices are main ingredients that can bring a vast change and provide a low-fat vegetarian recipe that is enjoyable and yummy.

A lot of recipes of low calorie vegetarian dishes can be found online. An individual can also purchase vegetarian cookery books with low-fat recipes in them. A more practical and an effortless method for making low calorie vegetarian recipes is to just alter usual recipes by using healthy replacements like diet cheeses or replacing plain yogurt for vinegary cream.

If an individual is creative, they will be amazed to discover that you can discover plenteous healthy vegetarian recipes and able utilize these recipes into one's diet that will balance their weight loss targets.

All a person requires is a little learning into where one can make replacements that will turn high calorie foods into light foods with a small amount of variation and numerous thoughts. Embrace low calorie vegan recipes into your daily diet plan and become conscious that you can consume tasty foods while sustaining your meatless standard of living.

VEGAN VEGETARIAN

The difference between vegetarian and non-vegetarian is widely understood as the eating habits are distinct and obvious.

There is another branch of food eating group commonly known as vegan and the difference between vegetarian and vegan is misunderstood. There is no striking difference between vegan and vegetarian eating habits but still people get confused in categorizing these food eating groups.

As a layman you will not be able to understand the difference between vegan and vegetarian. People consider these as same food eating groups because the similarities are obvious and clear.

People believe what they see and you often spot a vegetarian eating green fresh salads and few broccolis for all three meals. The fact is different vegans and vegetarians consume foods very differently and their ways are not always similar. Understanding the eating trends of this faction will make things clear.

Below few examples:

People who consume dairy products, eggs, fruits and vegetables are categorized as Lacto-ovo-vegetarian. It is one of the most recurrent and frequent type of lacto-vegetarian diet. There are cases where you find these groups eating fish and also consuming poultry products.

Lacto-vegetarian: Their diet includes vegetables, healthy nuts, fruits, grains and dairy products. The only difference is egg consumption which this group avoids.

Vegan: The difference between vegans and vegetarian can be understood by following their food habits. Vegans do not include dairy foodstuffs, eggs or any sort of animal products in their regular diet. Not only have these vegans refrained from sporting or wearing anything which is derived from animal products.

Macrobiotic: There are many reasons to follow a diet group. Diet which is followed on grounds of philosophy and spirituality is known as Macrobiotic diet. Health factors are also taken into account before selecting this diet. In this diet food is categorized as negative and positive food. The positive group is ying and negative is yang. There are levels of progression in this type of diet. The elimination of animal products is encouraged at all levels. The highest level eliminates even fruits and vegetables and is confined to brown rice.

A normal person will definitely get confused between the lacto-vegetarian and vegetarian diet. But for the vegans and vegetarian it is absolutely easy to follow their life style. It's only when you start to follow a diet regime you come to know the positives and negatives. You should support all diet groups and food eating habits as far as it's is healthy and keeps you strong.

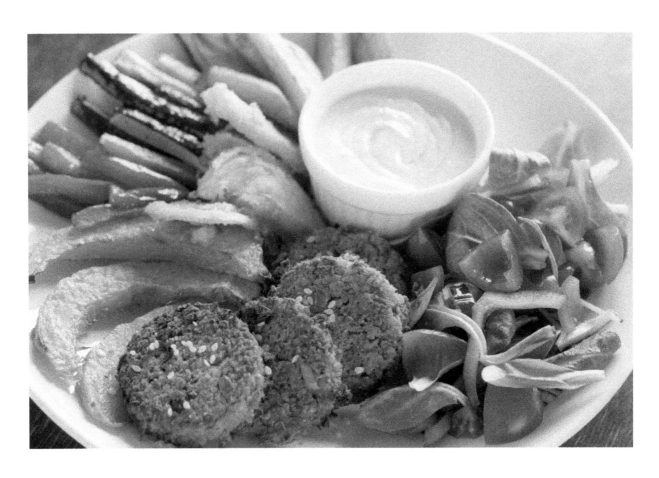

97 DELICIOUS
RECIPES

Easy Vegetarian Red Beans Lasagna

Ingredients

1 tablespoon olive oil
1 small onion, chopped
1 clove garlic, minced
1 (15 ounce) can red beans, drained
1 (14.5 ounce) can diced tomatoes, drained
1/2 red bell pepper, chopped
1 teaspoon dried basil
1 teaspoon dried oregano
salt and pepper to taste
3 tablespoons butter
3 tablespoons all-purpose flour
1 1/2 cups cold milk
1/2 cup grated Parmesan cheese
4 no-boil lasagna noodles
4 ounces shredded Gruyere cheese

Directions

Preheat oven to 350 degrees F (175 degrees C).

Heat the olive oil in a skillet over medium heat, and cook the onion until tender. Mix in garlic, and cook until heated through. Mix in red beans, tomatoes, and red bell pepper. Season with basil, oregano, salt, and pepper. Continue cooking 10 minutes, stirring occasionally.

Melt the butter in a saucepan over medium heat, and gradually mix in flour until smooth. Slowly stir in the milk. Mix in Parmesan cheese, and continue to cook and stir until slightly thickened.

Spread 1/2 the red bean mixture in a 9x9 inch casserole dish, and top with 2 lasagna noodles. Layer with remaining bean mixture and remaining noodles. Cover with the sauce, and top with Gruyere cheese.

Bake 20 minutes in the preheated oven, or until lightly browned.

Spicy Vegetarian Lasagna

Ingredients

1 (16 ounce) package lasagna noodles
2 teaspoons olive oil
2/3 cup diced red bell pepper
2/3 cup diced orange bell pepper
2/3 cup diced yellow bell pepper
2/3 cup diced green bell pepper
1 small yellow onion, diced
2 (14.5 ounce) cans diced tomatoes
1 (6 ounce) can tomato paste
1 1/2 cups water
1 dash crushed red pepper flakes
1/4 cup grated Parmesan cheese
1 (15 ounce) container ricotta cheese
1 (8 ounce) package shredded mozzarella cheese
4 eggs
1/4 teaspoon black pepper
1/4 teaspoon dried oregano, crushed
1/4 cup grated Parmesan cheese (optional)

Directions

Bring a large pot of lightly salted water to a boil. Cook lasagna pasta in boiling water for 8 to 10 minutes, or until al dente. Drain, rinse with cold water, and place on wax paper to cool.

Cook bell peppers and onion in olive oil in a large sauce pan until onions are translucent. Stir in diced tomatoes, tomato paste, water, and red pepper flakes. More red pepper flakes can be added if spicier sauce is preferred. Simmer for 30 minutes.

Preheat oven to 375 degrees F (190 degrees C). In a medium bowl, combine Parmesan cheese, ricotta cheese, mozzarella cheese, eggs, black pepper, and oregano.

Place a small amount of sauce in the bottom of a 9x13 inch baking dish. Reserve 1/2 cup of the sauce. Place three lasagna noodles lengthwise in pan. Layer some of the cheese mixture and the vegetable sauce on top of noodles. Repeat layering with remaining ingredients, ending with noodles. Spread reserved sauce over top of noodles. Sprinkle with grated Parmesan cheese, if desired.

Cover dish with foil, and bake for 40 minutes or until bubbly. Remove foil during last 10 minutes of baking.

Rae's Vegetarian Chili

Ingredients

4 cloves garlic, minced
2 tablespoons olive oil
1 (28 ounce) can diced tomatoes with juice
1 (8 ounce) can tomato sauce
1 (6 ounce) can tomato paste
1 (12 fluid ounce) can or bottle beer
4 tablespoons chili powder, or to taste
1 tablespoon mustard powder
1 teaspoon dried oregano
freshly ground black pepper
1 teaspoon ground cumin
1/8 teaspoon hot pepper sauce
1 (15 ounce) can black beans, rinsed and drained
1 (15 ounce) can garbanzo beans, drained
1 (15 ounce) can pinto beans, drained and rinsed
1 (15 ounce) can kidney beans, drained and rinsed
1 (15 ounce) can cannellini beans, drained and rinsed
1 (15 ounce) can whole kernel corn, drained and rinsed
2 cups shredded Cheddar cheese

Directions

In a 4 quart pot, saute garlic in oil.

Add diced tomatoes (undrained), tomato sauce, tomato paste, beer, chili powder, mustard powder, oregano, pepper, cumin, hot pepper sauce. Stir in the pinto beans, garbanzo beans, black beans, red and white kidney beans, and corn. Bring the mixture to a boil, reduce heat, and let simmer for 20 minutes. Top each serving with cheese (if you'd like).

Vegetarian Cabbage Rolls

Ingredients

1/3 cup uncooked brown rice
2/3 cup water
2 cups textured vegetable protein
3/4 cup boiling water
2 (10.75 ounce) cans tomato soup
10 3/4 fluid ounces water
1 large head cabbage, cored
1 tablespoon vegetable oil
1 large onion, chopped
1/2 carrot, finely chopped
1/2 red bell pepper, diced
3 cloves garlic, minced
1 tablespoon white wine
1 (14.5 ounce) can whole peeled tomatoes, drained, juice reserved
1 egg, lightly beaten
1/2 cup frozen peas
2 pinches cayenne pepper
1/2 teaspoon onion powder
1 teaspoon garlic powder
1/2 teaspoon dried basil
3 drops hot red pepper sauce
toothpicks
salt and pepper to taste

Directions

Place the rice and 2/3 cup water in a pot, and bring to a boil. Reduce heat to low, cover, and simmer 40 minutes, until tender. Mix the textured vegetable protein and 3/4 cup boiling water in a medium bowl. Soak 15 minutes, until rehydrated. Mix in the cooked rice.

Preheat oven to 350 degrees F (175 degrees C). In a bowl, mix the tomato soup and 10 3/4 fluid ounces (1 soup can) water.

Place the cabbage in a pot with enough water to cover. Bring to a boil, and cook 15 minutes, until leaves are easily removed. Drain, cool, and separate leaves.

Heat the oil in a skillet over medium heat. Stir in the onion, carrot, red bell pepper, and garlic. Cook until tender. Mix in wine, and continue cooking until almost all liquid has evaporated. Stir in rice and textured vegetable protein, reserved juice from the tomatoes, egg, and peas. Season with cayenne pepper, onion powder, garlic powder, basil, and hot pepper sauce. Cook and stir until heated through.

On 1 cabbage leaf, place about 2 tablespoons skillet mixture and 1 tomato. Roll tightly, and seal with a toothpick. Repeat with remaining filling. Arrange in a casserole dish. Pour the soup and water over cabbage rolls. Season with salt and pepper.

Cover, and bake 35 minutes in the preheated oven, basting occasionally with the tomato sauce. Remove cover, and continue baking 10 minutes.

Vegetarian Purple Potatoes with Onions and

Ingredients

6 purple potatoes, scrubbed
1 tablespoon olive oil
1 large red onion, chopped
8 ounces sliced fresh mushrooms
salt and black pepper to taste
2 tablespoons olive oil
1/4 teaspoon crushed red pepper flakes
1 tablespoon chopped capers
1 teaspoon chopped fresh tarragon

Directions

Cut each potato into wedges by quartering the potatoes, then cutting each quarter in half. Heat 1 tablespoon of olive oil over medium heat in a large skillet, and cook and stir the onion and mushrooms until the mushrooms start to release their liquid and the onion becomes translucent, about 5 minutes. Transfer the onion and mushrooms into a bowl, and set aside.

Heat 2 more tablespoons of olive oil over high heat in the same skillet, and place the potato wedges into the hot oil. Sprinkle with salt and pepper, and allow to cook, stirring occasionally, until the wedges are browned on both sides, about 10 minutes. Reduce heat to medium, sprinkle the potato wedges with red pepper flakes, and allow to cook until the potatoes are tender, about 10 more minutes. Stir in the onion and mushroom mixture, toss the vegetables together, and mix in the capers and fresh tarragon.

Vegetarian Carrot Cake

Ingredients

3 teaspoons lemon juice
1 1/4 cups milk
2/3 cup vegetable oil
2 teaspoons orange zest
3/4 cup packed brown sugar
3 teaspoons vanilla extract
1 1/2 cups whole wheat flour
1 1/2 cups all-purpose flour
1 1/2 teaspoons baking powder
1 1/2 teaspoons ground cinnamon
1/2 teaspoon ground cloves
1/2 teaspoon salt
1 1/2 cups grated carrots
1/2 cup chopped walnuts

Directions

Preheat oven to 350 degrees F (175 degrees C). Butter an 8 inch springform pan. In a small bowl, add lemon juice to milk. Stir together and let stand 5 minutes. Sift flour, baking powder, cinnamon, cloves and salt together and set aside.

In a large bowl, cream oil, orange zest and brown sugar. Add sour milk and vanilla. Add flour mixture and beat until smooth. Stir in the grated carrots and chopped nuts.

Pour the batter into an 8 inch springform or other deep 8 inch pan. Bake at 350 degrees F (175 degrees C) for 1 hour, or until a toothpick inserted into the cake comes out clean. Allow to cool.

Vegetarian Penne

Ingredients

2 cups uncooked penne or medium tube pasta
1/3 cup finely chopped onion
1 small yellow summer squash, sliced
1 small zucchini, sliced
1/2 cup sliced fresh mushrooms
1 teaspoon minced garlic
3 tablespoons butter
1 tablespoon all-purpose flour
1/2 teaspoon salt
1/4 teaspoon dried parsley flakes
1/4 teaspoon dried thyme
1/4 teaspoon pepper
1/4 cup heavy whipping cream

Directions

Cook pasta according to package directions. Meanwhile, in a large skillet, saute the onion, summer squash, zucchini, mushrooms and garlic in butter until tender.

In a bowl, whisk the flour, seasonings and cream until smooth; add to the skillet. Cook for 2-3 minutes or until thickened. Drain pasta and add to vegetable mixture. Cook for 2-3 minutes or until heated through.

Ingredients

1 (15.5 ounce) can great northern beans, rinsed and drained
2 cups hot cooked angel hair pasta
3 tablespoons butter or margarine
1/4 teaspoon garlic salt
1/4 cup shredded Parmesan or Romano cheese
Minced fresh parsley

Directions

Place beans in a microwave-safe dish; cover and microwave on high for 2 minutes or until heated through. Place pasta in a serving bowl. Add butter and garlic salt if desired; toss until butter is melted. Add beans and cheese; toss to coat. Sprinkle with parsley. Serve immediately.

One Dish Vegetarian Dinner

Ingredients

1 (16 ounce) package penne pasta
4 cloves garlic, minced
3/4 cup olive oil
1 large head fresh broccoli, blanched
1 (6 ounce) can sliced black olives

Directions

Cook pasta in large pot with boiling salted water until al dente. Drain well.

In a medium skillet over medium heat cook garlic in olive oil, being careful not to allow garlic to burn.

In a large bowl add the cooked broccoli, cooked and drained pasta, and black olives.

To serve, pour garlic oil over pasta and vegetables. Serve warm.

Vegetarian Quiche

Ingredients

1 (9 inch) unbaked pastry shell
1 1/2 cups chopped onion
1 medium green pepper, chopped
1 cup chopped tomatoes
1/2 cup chopped zucchini
1/2 cup sliced fresh mushrooms
2 tablespoons butter or margarine
1/4 teaspoon curry powder
1/2 teaspoon salt
1/4 teaspoon pepper
Pinch ground cinnamon
5 eggs
1/4 cup milk
1/4 cup grated Parmesan cheese

Directions

Line unpricked pastry shell with a double thickness of heavy-duty foil. Bake at 450 degrees F for 5 minutes. Remove foil; bake 5 minutes longer. Reduce heat to 350 degrees F.

In a skillet, saute the onion, green pepper, tomatoes, zucchini and mushrooms in butter. Add the curry powder, salt, pepper and cinnamon; mix well. Spoon into crust.

In a bowl, beat eggs. Add the milk and cheese; mix well. Carefully pour over vegetables. Bake for 40-45 minutes or until a knife inserted near the center comes out clean. Let stand for 5 minutes before cutting.

Italian Vegetarian Patties

Ingredients

2 tablespoons vegetable oil
3/4 cup uncooked brown rice
1 1/2 cups red lentils
6 cups water
1 teaspoon salt
2 eggs
2 1/2 cups dry bread crumbs
1 1/2 cups grated Parmesan cheese
2 teaspoons dried basil
1 1/2 teaspoons garlic powder
3 tablespoons vegetable oil

Directions

Heat 2 tablespoons oil in a large saucepan. Stir in the brown rice, and cook until golden brown. Add the lentils, water, and salt; bring to a boil. Reduce heat to low, cover, and cook until the rice is tender and the water is absorbed, about 40 minutes. Add additional water if needed; mixture should be very thick. Remove from heat and let cool slightly.

Place the cooked rice mixture in a food processor along with the eggs, bread crumbs, Parmesan cheese, basil, and garlic powder. Process until well combined, and the texture of ground meat. Form into 1/4 to 1/2 inch thick patties, using about 3 tablespoons mixture for each.

Heat 3 tablespoons oil in a large skillet. In batches, fry patties until browned, about 2 to 3 minutes per side. Drain on paper towels; cool. Fry remaining patties in the same manner. Store in airtight containers in the refrigerator or freezer.

Vegetarian Black Bean Chili

Ingredients

1/2 cup applesauce
1 tablespoon brown sugar
1 tablespoon ground coriander
1 teaspoon ground cayenne pepper
1 teaspoon ground cumin
1 teaspoon dried oregano 1/2 teaspoon ground cloves 1/2 teaspoon dried rosemary 1/2 teaspoon dried sage
1/4 teaspoon dried thyme
1 pinch asafoetida powder (optional)
1 (15 ounce) can black beans
1 (6 ounce) can tomato paste
2 cloves garlic, minced
1 onion, chopped
1 yellow squash, chopped
2 carrots, chopped
1 sweet potato, peeled and diced
1 cup chopped fresh mushrooms
1 quart water, or as needed

Directions

In a large pot over medium-low heat, mix the applesauce, brown sugar, coriander, cayenne pepper, cumin, oregano, cloves, rosemary, sage, thyme and asafoetida powder. Cook just until heated through. Stir in black beans and tomato paste. Mix in garlic, onion, squash, carrots, sweet potato and mushrooms. Pour in enough water to cover. Bring to a boil, reduce heat to low and simmer 45 minutes, stirring occasionally.

Vegetarian Bean Curry

Ingredients

2 tablespoons olive oil
1 large white onion, chopped
1/2 cup dry lentils
2 cloves garlic, minced
3 tablespoons curry powder
1 teaspoon ground cumin
1 pinch cayenne pepper
1 (28 ounce) can crushed tomatoes
1 (15 ounce) can garbanzo beans, drained and rinsed
1 (8 ounce) can kidney beans, drained and rinsed
1/2 cup raisins
salt and pepper to taste

Directions

Heat the oil in a large pot over medium heat, and cook the onion until tender. Mix in the lentils and garlic, and season with curry powder, cumin, and cayenne pepper. Cook and stir 2 minutes. Stir in the tomatoes, garbanzo beans, kidney beans, and raisins. Season with salt and pepper. Reduce heat to low, and simmer at least 1 hour, stirring occasionally.

Vegetarian Cake

Ingredients

2 cups all-purpose flour
1 tablespoon baking powder
1 1/2 teaspoons ground cinnamon
1 1/2 teaspoons ground allspice
3/4 teaspoon baking soda
1/4 teaspoon salt
1 1/2 cups peeled and shredded apples
1 1/2 cups shredded carrots
1 1/2 cups peeled and shredded potatoes
3/4 cup dried currants
3/4 cup raisins
3/4 cup chopped walnuts
1 tablespoon grated orange zest
3/4 cup butter, softened
1 1/2 cups brown sugar
3 eggs
2 tablespoons light molasses

Directions

Preheat oven to 350 degrees F (175 degrees C). Grease and flour a 10-inch bundt pan.

Onto a sheet of waxed paper, sift flour, baking powder, cinnamon, allspice, baking soda and salt. Set aside. In a medium bowl, stir together apples, carrots, potatoes, currants, raisins, walnuts and orange zest. Set aside.

Place softened butter and brown sugar in a large mixing bowl. Beat at low speed until mixture is light and fluffy. Add eggs one at a time, beating after each addition, and then mix in molasses. Slowly beat in dry ingredients until mixture is thoroughly moistened. Gradually stir in fruit mixture and continue to beat at low speed until well blended. Spoon into prepared pan.

Bake in preheated oven for 60 minutes, or until a toothpick inserted in center comes out clean and cake pulls away from sides of pan. Cool on a wire rack for 10 minutes, then remove from pan and cool completely.

Lucie's Vegetarian Chili

Ingredients

1/3 cup olive oil
2 cups chopped onion
3/4 cup chopped celery
1 cup chopped green bell pepper
1 cup chopped carrots
1 tablespoon minced garlic
2 cups chopped mushrooms
1/4 teaspoon crushed red pepper flakes
1 tablespoon ground cumin
2 tablespoons chili powder
3/4 teaspoon dried basil
2 teaspoons salt
1/2 teaspoon ground black pepper

2 cups tomato juice
3/4 cup bulgur wheat
2 cups chopped tomatoes
1 (20 ounce) can kidney beans, undrained
1/2 teaspoon hot pepper sauce (such as Tabasco®)
2 tablespoons lemon juice
3 tablespoons tomato paste
1 tablespoon Worcestershire sauce
1/4 cup dry red wine
2 tablespoons canned chopped green chile peppers, or to taste

Directions

Heat the olive oil in a large pot over high heat. Stir in the onion, celery, green bell pepper, carrot, garlic, mushrooms, red pepper flakes, cumin, chili powder, basil, salt, and pepper. Cook and stir until the vegetables begin to soften, about 2 minutes. Stir in the tomato juice, bulgur wheat, chopped tomatoes, kidney beans, hot pepper sauce, lemon juice, tomato paste, Worcestershire sauce, red wine, and green chile peppers. Bring to a boil, stirring frequently. Reduce heat to medium-low, and simmer, uncovered, 20 minutes before serving.

Vegetarian Lime Orzo

Ingredients

2 tablespoons olive oil
2 cloves garlic, minced
2 cups orzo pasta
1 zucchini, peeled and shredded
1 carrot, peeled and shredded
1 (16 ounce) can stewed tomatoes, undrained
1 (14 ounce) can vegetable broth
1 teaspoon Italian seasoning
1 teaspoon dried basil leaves
salt and black pepper to taste
1/4 cup chopped green onions
1/4 cup chopped fresh parsley
2 teaspoons grated lime zest
2 tablespoons lime juice
1/2 cup grated Parmesan cheese for topping

Directions

Heat the olive oil in a large skillet over medium-high heat. Stir in the garlic and orzo pasta; cook and stir until pasta turns a light, golden color, about 5 minutes. Stir in zucchini and carrots; cook until vegetables soften, about 2 minutes. Stir in the tomatoes, vegetable broth, Italian seasoning, and basil. Season with salt and pepper to taste. Reduce heat to medium. Cover, and simmer until almost all liquid is absorbed, about 10 minutes. Stir in the green onions, parsley, lime zest, and lime juice. Remove from heat, cool slightly, and serve sprinkled with Parmesan cheese.

Vegetarian Sweet and Sour Meatballs

Ingredients

Meatballs:
4 eggs
1 cup shredded Cheddar cheese
1/2 cup cottage cheese
1/2 cup finely chopped onion
1 cup finely chopped pecans
1 teaspoon dried basil
1 1/2 teaspoons salt
1/4 teaspoon dried sage
2 cups Italian seasoned bread crumbs
Sweet and Sour Sauce:
1/4 cup vegetable oil
1/4 cup white vinegar
3/4 cup apricot jam
1 cup ketchup
1/4 cup minced onion
1 teaspoon dried oregano
1 dash hot pepper sauce

Directions

Preheat the oven to 350 degrees F (175 degrees C).

In a large bowl, mix together the eggs, Cheddar cheese, and cottage cheese until well blended. Mix in 1/2 cup onion, pecans, basil, salt and sage. Stir in bread crumbs. Form the mixture into 2 inch balls, and place them in a 9x13 inch baking dish.

In another bowl, whisk together the vegetable oil, vinegar, apricot jam, ketchup, 1/4 cup onion, oregano and hot pepper sauce. Pour over meatballs.

Bake uncovered for 35 to 40 minutes in the preheated oven, until meatballs are firm, and sauce is thick and bubbly.

Vegetarian Meatloaf

Ingredients

1 (12 ounce) bottle barbeque sauce
1 (12 ounce) package vegetarian burger crumbles
1 green bell pepper, chopped
1/3 cup minced onion
1 clove garlic, minced
1/2 cup soft bread crumbs
3 tablespoons Parmesan cheese
1 egg, beaten
1/4 teaspoon dried thyme
1/4 teaspoon dried basil
1/4 teaspoon parsley flakes
salt and pepper to taste

Directions

Preheat oven to 325 degrees F (165 degrees C). Lightly grease a 5x9 inch loaf pan.

In a bowl, mix 1/2 the barbeque sauce with the vegetarian burger crumbles, green bell pepper, onion, garlic, bread crumbs, Parmesan cheese, and egg. Season with thyme, basil, parsley, salt, and pepper. Transfer to the loaf pan.

Bake 45 minutes in the preheated oven. Pour remaining barbeque sauce over the loaf, and continue baking 15 minutes, or until loaf is set.

Vegetarian Stuffed Peppers

Ingredients

1 1/2 cups brown rice
6 large green bell peppers
3 tablespoons soy sauce
3 tablespoons cooking sherry
1 teaspoon vegetarian Worcestershire sauce
1 1/2 cups extra firm tofu
1/2 cup sweetened dried cranberries
1/4 cup chopped pecans
1/2 cup grated Parmesan cheese
salt and pepper to taste
2 cups tomato sauce
2 tablespoons brown sugar

Directions

Preheat oven to 350 degrees F (175 degrees C). In a saucepan bring 3 cups water to a boil. Stir in rice. Reduce heat, cover and simmer for 40 minutes.

Meanwhile, core and seed green peppers, leaving bottoms intact. Place peppers in a microwavable dish with about 1/2 inch of water in the bottom. Microwave on high for 6 minutes.

In a small frying pan bring soy sauce, wine and Worcestershire sauce to a simmer. Add tofu and simmer until the liquid is absorbed. Combine rice (after it has cooled), tofu, cranberries, nuts, cheese, salt and pepper; mix and pack firmly into peppers. Return peppers to the dish you first microwaved them in, and bake in preheated oven for 25 to 30 minutes, or until lightly browned on top.

Meanwhile, in a small saucepan over low heat, combine tomato sauce and brown sugar; heat until hot throughout. Spoon sauce over each serving.

Vegetarian's Delight Pizza

Ingredients

1 (12 inch) pre-baked pizza crust
2 tablespoons olive oil
1 cup seasoned tomato sauce
1/2 cup sliced onion
1 cup fresh sliced mushrooms
1/2 cup chopped green bell pepper
1/4 cup chopped black olives
2 cups shredded mozzarella cheese

Directions

Preheat the oven to 350 degrees F (175 degrees C).

Place the pizza crust on a large cookie tray or pizza pan. Brush the crust evenly with olive oil. Spread tomato sauce over it with a spatula or back of a spoon. Sprinkle vegetables evenly over the sauce, and top with cheese.

Bake for 10 to 12 minutes, or until cheese has melted and is bubbly. Let cool for 2 to 3 minutes before cutting.

Vegetarian Meatloaf with Vegetables

Ingredients

1/2 (14 ounce) package vegetarian ground beef (e.g., Gimme Lean TM)
1 (12 ounce) package vegetarian burger crumbles
1 onion, chopped
2 eggs, beaten
2 tablespoons vegetarian Worcestershire sauce
1 teaspoon salt
1/3 teaspoon pepper
1 teaspoon ground sage
1/2 teaspoon garlic powder
2 teaspoons prepared mustard
1 tablespoon vegetable oil
3 1/2 slices bread, cubed
1/3 cup milk
1 (8 ounce) can tomato sauce
4 carrots, cut into 1 inch pieces
4 potatoes, cubed
1 cooking spray

Directions

Preheat oven to 350 degrees F (175 degrees C).

In a large bowl combine vegetarian ground beef, vegetarian ground beef crumbles, onion, eggs, Worcestershire sauce, salt, pepper, sage, garlic powder, mustard, oil, bread cubes and milk. Transfer to a 9 x 13 inch baking dish and form into a loaf. Pour tomato sauce on top.

Place carrots and potatoes around loaf and spray vegetables with cooking spray.

Bake 30 to 45 minutes; turn vegetables. Bake another 30 to 45 minutes. Let stand 15 minutes before slicing.

Vegetarian Baked Pasta

Ingredients

1 pound penne pasta
2 tablespoons olive oil
8 ounces portobello mushrooms, cut into 1/2 inch pieces
1 teaspoon dried basil
1 teaspoon dried oregano
2 cloves garlic, minced
1 (28 ounce) jar spaghetti sauce
4 cups shredded mozzarella cheese
8 ounces Gorgonzola cheese, crumbled

Directions

Bring a large pot of lightly salted water to a boil. Add pasta and cook for 8 to 10 minutes or until al dente; drain. Pour a glass of ice water over the pasta to stop the cooking, but do not rinse thoroughly.

Preheat oven to 350 degrees F (175 degrees C). Coat a 9 x 13 glass pan with olive oil. Heat 2 tablespoons olive oil in large skillet. Add mushrooms. Cook for 2 minutes then add basil, oregano and garlic and cook 1 minute more. Add sauce to mushroom mixture and stir.

To assemble, pour enough sauce in the bottom of the pan to cover. Combine the remaining sauce and the pasta. Place one-third of sauced noodles on top of sauce in pan. Top with 1 cup of mozzarella and one-half of the gorgonzola. Repeat for a second layer. Put the final third of the noodles in the pan and top with the final 2 cups of mozzarella.

Bake for 30 to 45 minutes, or until cheese is browned. Serve.

Vegetarian Refried Beans

Ingredients

1 pound dry pinto beans, rinsed
2 tablespoons minced garlic, divided
1 medium tomato, diced
2 tablespoons ground cumin
1 tablespoon chili powder
2 tablespoons olive oil
salt to taste

Directions

Place the beans in a large saucepan, and cover with an inch of water. Place over high heat, and bring to a boil. When the beans have come to a boil, drain, and return them to the same pot. Cover the beans with 2 inches of water, and stir in 1 tablespoon of garlic, the tomato, cumin, and chili powder. Bring to a boil over high heat, then reduce heat to low, and simmer until the beans are very soft, about 3 hours and 45 minutes, adding water as needed.

Once the beans have cooked, mash them with the remaining tablespoon of garlic, the oil, and salt to taste; use additional water as needed to achieve desired consistency. Place over low heat for 30 minutes, stirring occasionally. Serve.

Vegetarian Tortilla Soup

Ingredients

2 tablespoons vegetable oil
1 (1 pound) package frozen pepper and onion stir fry mix
2 cloves garlic, minced
3 tablespoons ground cumin
1 (28 ounce) can crushed tomatoes
3 (4 ounce) cans chopped green chile peppers, drained
4 (14 ounce) cans vegetable broth
salt and pepper to taste
1 (11 ounce) can whole kernel corn
12 ounces tortilla chips
1 cup shredded Cheddar cheese
1 avocado - peeled, pitted and diced

Directions

Heat the oil in a large pot over medium heat. Stir in the pepper and onion stir fry mix, garlic, and cumin, and cook 5 minutes, until vegetables are tender. Mix in the tomatoes and chile peppers. Pour in the broth, and season with salt and pepper. Bring to a boil, reduce heat to low, and simmer 30 minutes.

Mix corn into the soup, and continue cooking 5 minutes. Serve in bowls over equal amounts of tortilla chips. Top with cheese and avocado.

Vegetarian Four Cheese Lasagna

Ingredients

2 cups peeled and diced pumpkin
1 eggplant, sliced into 1/2 inch rounds
5 tomatoes
1 pint ricotta cheese
9 ounces crumbled feta cheese
2/3 cup pesto
2 eggs, beaten
salt and pepper to taste
1 (15 ounce) can tomato sauce
fresh pasta sheets
1 1/3 cups shredded mozzarella cheese
1 cup grated Parmesan cheese

Directions

Preheat oven to 350 degrees F (175 degrees C).

Place pumpkin on a baking sheet and roast in oven until browned and tender, about 30 minutes. Meanwhile, grill eggplant on a charcoal grill or fry in a skillet, turning once, until charred and tender, 10 to 15 minutes. Halve tomatoes and place on baking sheet in oven for last 15 minutes of pumpkin time; cook until tender and wrinkly.

In a medium bowl, stir together ricotta, feta, pesto, eggs, salt and pepper until well mixed. Fold roasted pumpkin into ricotta mixture.

Spoon half of the tomato sauce into a 9x13 baking dish. Lay two pasta sheets over the sauce. Arrange a single layer of eggplant slices over pasta and top with half the ricotta mixture. Cover with two more pasta sheets.   Arrange the roasted tomatoes evenly over the sheets and spoon the remaining half the ricotta mixture over the tomatoes. Sprinkle with half the mozzarella. Top with remaining two sheets of pasta. Pour remaining tomato sauce over all and sprinkle with remaining mozzarella and Parmesan.

Bake in preheated oven 30 to 40 minutes, until golden and bubbly.

Vegetarian Tortilla Stew

Ingredients

1 (19 ounce) can green enchilada sauce
1 1/2 cups water
1 cube vegetable bouillon
1/2 teaspoon garlic powder
1/4 teaspoon chili powder
1/4 teaspoon ground cumin
1 (15 ounce) can pinto beans, drained and rinsed
1/2 (16 ounce) can diced tomatoes
1 cup frozen corn
1/2 cup vegetarian chicken substitute, diced (optional)
4 (6 inch) corn tortillas, torn into strips
1 tablespoon chopped fresh cilantro
salt and pepper to taste

Directions

In a pot, mix the enchilada sauce and water. Dissolve the bouillon cube in the liquid, and season with garlic powder, chile powder, and cumin. Bring to a boil, and reduce heat to low. Mix in the beans, tomatoes, and corn. Simmer until heated through. Mix in vegetarian chicken and tortillas, and cook until heated through. Stir in cilantro, and season with salt and pepper to serve.

Vegetarian Moroccan Stew

Ingredients

1 tablespoon olive oil
1 yellow onion, diced
4 cloves garlic, minced
2 teaspoons ground cumin
1 (4 inch) cinnamon stick
salt and pepper to taste
1 pound butternut squash - peeled, seeded, and cut into 2-inch cubes
4 large red potatoes, cut into 2-inch cubes
2 cups vegetable broth
1 (15 ounce) can garbanzo beans, drained
1 (14.5 ounce) can canned diced tomatoes with their juice
1 cup pitted, brine-cured green olives
1/2 teaspoon lemon zest
1 3/4 cups water
1 (10 ounce) box uncooked couscous
6 tablespoons plain yogurt
6 tablespoons chopped fresh cilantro

Directions

Heat olive oil in a large covered saucepan or Dutch oven over medium heat, until oil is hot but not smoking. Drop in the onion, garlic, cumin, cinnamon stick, and salt and pepper. Cook and stir for 5 minutes, until onion is tender and translucent.

Stir in the butternut squash and potato cubes, broth, garbanzo beans, and tomatoes, and bring the mixture to a boil. Reduce heat, cover the pot, and simmer about 20 minutes, stirring occasionally, until the squash and potatoes are tender. Remove the stew from heat, and stir in the olives and lemon zest.

In a large saucepan, bring 1 3/4 cup water to a boil. Stir in couscous. Cover and remove from the heat; let stand for 5 minutes. Fluff with a fork; cool. Serve stew over cooked couscous. Garnish each serving with a dollop of yogurt and a sprinkle of cilantro leaves.

Vegetarian Faux Chicken Patties

Ingredients

1 (12.5 ounce) can vegetarian fried chicken (e.g., FriChik)
1 celery
1/2 small onion
1/4 large green bell pepper
4 eggs, beaten
1/2 cup dry bread stuffing mix
salt and pepper to taste
1 tablespoon olive oil

Directions

Process the 'chicken' in a food processor and then transfer it to a medium mixing bowl. Run the celery, onion and green pepper through the processor. Add the vegetables to the mixing bowl and stir in the eggs, stuffing, salt and pepper; mix well. Form into patties.

In a medium frying pan heat olive oil over medium-high heat. Fry patties on each side until browned.

Easy Vegetarian Corn Chowder

Ingredients

6 tablespoons butter
1/4 cup diced onion
1/2 cup diced celery
6 tablespoons all-purpose flour
2 (14.5 ounce) cans vegetable broth
2 (15 ounce) cans creamed corn
1 (15 ounce) can whole kernel corn, drained
2 tablespoons shredded carrot
1 cup half-and-half cream
3/4 cup skim milk
1/2 teaspoon ground nutmeg
1/4 teaspoon ground black pepper
1 pinch salt

Directions

In a large saucepan over medium heat, melt butter. Cook onions and celery in butter 3 minutes. Whisk in flour and cook 6 minutes more, until light brown. Whisk in broth and simmer 10 minutes.

Stir in creamed corn, corn, carrot, half-and-half, milk, nutmeg, pepper and salt. Simmer over low heat 10 minutes more.

Nut Burgers (Vegetarian)

Ingredients

1/2 cup finely chopped walnuts
1/2 cup unsalted sunflower seeds
1 cup canned chickpeas, drained
1/4 cup diced red onion
1 beaten egg
1 tablespoon chopped fresh parsley
1/4 teaspoon fresh ground black pepper
1 tablespoon salt-free herb seasoning blend
2 tablespoons olive oil
2 slices mild Cheddar cheese
1 pita bread round
1/4 cup prepared Ranch salad dressing
2 leaves romaine lettuce
1 medium tomato, thinly sliced
1/2 avocado - peeled, pitted and sliced

Directions

Place walnuts and sunflower seeds in a dry skillet over medium heat. Cook, stirring occasionally until lightly toasted and fragrant, about 5 minutes.

In a medium bowl, mash garbanzo beans with a fork, or chop in a food processor. Stir in the onion, egg, parsley, and toasted nuts. Season with pepper and seasoning blend, and mix well.

Heat olive oil in a skillet over medium heat. Divide the bean mixture into 2 patties, and fry in the hot oil for about 3 minutes on each side, or until well browned and heated through. Place a slice of cheese over each patty, and remove from heat.

Place the pita round in the same dry skillet the nuts were in, and heat for about 1 minute on each side. Cut the round in half, spread ranch dressing inside of each, and line the pockets with romaine leaves. Place a cheesy patty into each one, and top with sliced tomato and avocado. Serve with tortilla or potato chips.

Vegetarian Brown Rice Casserole

Ingredients

1 (19 ounce) can ready-to-serve lentil soup
1 cup cooked brown rice
1 (7.75 ounce) can unsalted mixed vegetables, drained
1 large canned roasted red pepper, diced
1/2 cup shredded sharp Cheddar cheese, divided

Directions

Combine soup, rice, mixed vegetables, peppers and 6 tablespoons of the cheddar cheese in a 2-quart, microwave-safe casserole or baking dish. Season with salt and pepper to taste, and level the top of the mixture. Sprinkle with the remaining 2 tablespoons of cheddar cheese.

Cover and cook in a microwave oven at full power until heated through and the cheese has melted (about 5 minutes).

Uncover and cool for 1 minute before serving.

Hariton's 'Famous' Vegetarian Casserole

Ingredients

8 large eggplants
8 large potatoes
8 green bell peppers
8 large onions
8 summer squash
6 tomatoes
1 pound fresh green beans
1 pound whole fresh mushrooms
2 bulbs garlic, cloves separated and peeled
1/4 cup chopped fresh dill weed
1/4 cup chopped fresh oregano
1/4 cup chopped fresh basil
1 (15 ounce) can tomato sauce
3/4 cup olive oil
salt and pepper to taste

Directions

Prepare the eggplant before assembling ingredients, by cutting them into 2 inch chunks and putting them into an extra large bowl with salted water to cover. This will draw out the bitterness from the eggplant. Let this sit for about 3 hours.

Preheat oven to 375 degrees F (190 degrees C).

Cut the potatoes, green bell peppers, onion, squash and tomatoes into 2-inch chunks. Cut the green beans and mushrooms in half and peel the garlic cloves.

Drain and rinse the eggplant, then combine it with all the other chopped vegetables, the dill, oregano and basil and place all into a 3x13x18 inch roasting pan. Pour the tomato sauce and olive oil over all.

Bake at 375 degrees F (190 degrees C) for 2 1/2 hours, adding a little water about halfway through cooking time to keep moist.

Vegetarian Shepherd's Pie II

Ingredients

2 cups vegetable broth, divided
1 teaspoon yeast extract spread,
e.g. Marmite/Vegemite
1/2 cup dry lentils
1/4 cup pearl barley
1 large carrot, diced
1/2 onion, finely chopped
1/2 cup walnuts, coarsely
chopped
3 potatoes, chopped
1 teaspoon all-purpose flour
1/2 teaspoon water
salt and pepper to taste

Directions

Preheat oven to 350 degrees F (175 degrees C).

In a large saucepan over medium-low heat, combine 1 1/4 cups broth, yeast extract, lentils and barley. Simmer for 30 minutes.

Meanwhile, in a medium saucepan combine remaining 3/4 cup broth, carrot, onion and walnuts; cook until tender, about 15 minutes.

Meanwhile, bring a large pot of salted water to a boil. Add potatoes and cook until tender but still firm, about 15 minutes. Drain and mash.

Combine flour and water and stir into carrot mixture; simmer until thickened. Combine carrot mixture with lentil mixture and season with salt and pepper. Pour mixture into a 2 quart casserole dish. Spoon mashed potatoes over lentil mixture.

Bake in preheated oven until lightly browned on top, about 30 minutes.

Unbelievably Easy and Delicious Vegetarian Chili

Ingredients

1 (28 ounce) can diced tomatoes with juice
1 small onion, diced
1 (15 ounce) can white beans, drained
1 (15 ounce) can chili beans, with liquid
1 (1.25 ounce) package reduced sodium taco seasoning mix
1 (1 ounce) package ranch dressing mix
1 (12 ounce) package vegetarian burger crumbles
1 (8 ounce) package shredded Cheddar cheese (optional)

Directions

Mix the tomatoes, onion, white beans, chili beans, taco seasoning mix, and ranch dressing mix in a large pot over medium heat. Bring to a boil. Reduce heat to low, mix in the burger crumbles, and continue cooking until heated through. Top with cheese to serve.

Veggie Vegetarian Chili

Ingredients

1 tablespoon vegetable oil
3 cloves garlic, minced
1 cup chopped onion
1 cup chopped carrots
1 cup chopped green bell pepper
1 cup chopped red bell pepper
2 tablespoons chili powder
1 1/2 cups chopped fresh mushrooms
1 (28 ounce) can whole peeled tomatoes with liquid, chopped
1 (15 ounce) can black beans, undrained
1 (15 ounce) can kidney beans, undrained
1 (15 ounce) can pinto beans, undrained
1 (15 ounce) can whole kernel corn, drained
1 tablespoon cumin
1 1/2 tablespoons dried oregano
1 1/2 tablespoons dried basil
1/2 tablespoon garlic powder

Directions

Heat the oil in a large pot over medium heat. Cook and stir the garlic, onion, and carrots in the pot until tender. Mix in the green bell pepper and red bell pepper. Season with chili powder. Continue cooking 5 minutes, or until peppers are tender.

Mix the mushrooms into the pot. Stir in the tomatoes with liquid, black beans with liquid, kidney beans with liquid, pinto beans with liquid, and corn. Season with cumin, oregano, basil, and garlic powder. Bring to a boil. Reduce heat to medium, cover, and cook 20 minutes, stirring occasionally.

Vegetarian Jambalaya

Ingredients

1 medium onion, finely chopped
1 cup chopped celery
1 cup chopped green pepper
1 cup sliced fresh mushrooms
2 garlic cloves, minced
1 teaspoon olive oil
3 cups chopped fresh tomatoes
2 cups water
1 cup uncooked long grain rice
2 tablespoons reduced-sodium soy sauce
1 tablespoon minced fresh parsley
1/4 teaspoon salt
1/4 teaspoon paprika
1/8 teaspoon cayenne pepper
1/8 teaspoon chili powder
1/8 teaspoon pepper
6 tablespoons reduced fat sour cream

Directions

In a large nonstick skillet, saute the onion, celery, green pepper, mushrooms and garlic in oil until tender. Stir in the tomatoes, water, rice, soy sauce, parsley, salt, paprika, cayenne, chili powder and pepper.

Transfer to a 2-1/2-qt. baking dish coated with nonstick cooking spray. Cover and bake at 350 degrees F for 65-70 minutes or until rice is tender and liquid is absorbed. Top each serving with 1 tablespoon sour cream.

Southwestern Vegetarian Pasta

Ingredients

1 tablespoon vegetable oil
1 onion, chopped
1/2 green bell pepper, diced
2 cloves garlic, chopped
2 tablespoons chili powder
1 teaspoon ground cumin
1 (28 ounce) can diced tomatoes with juice
1 (15 ounce) can chickpeas
1 (10 ounce) package frozen corn kernels, thawed
1 (12 ounce) package uncooked elbow macaroni
1/2 cup shredded Monterey Jack cheese

Directions

Heat oil in a large, deep skillet. Saute onion, green pepper, garlic, chili powder and cumin. Stir in tomatoes, chickpeas and corn. Reduce heat to low and simmer 15 to 20 minutes, or until thickened and heated through.

Meanwhile, bring a large pot of lightly salted water to a boil. Add macaroni and cook for 8 to 10 minutes or until al dente; drain.

Combine pasta and sauce. Sprinkle each serving with Monterey Jack cheese.

Vegetarian Stuffing

Ingredients

1 (1 pound) loaf day-old bread
1 (10.75 ounce) can condensed cream of mushroom soup
1 (10.5 ounce) can vegetable broth
1/4 cup water
1 teaspoon poultry seasoning
salt to taste
ground black pepper to taste
1/2 cup wild rice, cooked (optional)
1/4 cup dried cranberries (optional)
1/2 cup chopped mushrooms (optional)
1/4 cup chopped walnuts (optional)
1/4 cup cubed apples (optional)

Directions

Mix together the bread, cream of mushroom soup, vegetable broth, water, poultry seasoning, and salt and pepper to taste. Add any or all of the optional ingredients as desired. It will be sticky. Shape into a loaf and wrap in (nonstick, sprayed) foil to bake.

Bake for about an hour at 350 degrees F (175 degrees C). You can slice it like a meatloaf and serve.

Insanely Easy Vegetarian Chili

Ingredients

1 tablespoon vegetable oil
1 cup chopped onions
3/4 cup chopped carrots
3 cloves garlic, minced
1 cup chopped green bell pepper
1 cup chopped red bell pepper
3/4 cup chopped celery
1 tablespoon chili powder
1 1/2 cups chopped fresh mushrooms
1 (28 ounce) can whole peeled tomatoes with liquid, chopped
1 (19 ounce) can kidney beans with liquid
1 (11 ounce) can whole kernel corn, undrained
1 tablespoon ground cumin
1 1/2 teaspoons dried oregano
1 1/2 teaspoons dried basil

Directions

Heat oil in a large saucepan over medium heat. Saute onions, carrots, and garlic until tender. Stir in green pepper, red pepper, celery, and chili powder. Cook until vegetables are tender, about 6 minutes.

Stir in mushrooms, and cook 4 minutes. Stir in tomatoes, kidney beans, and corn. Season with cumin, oregano, and basil. Bring to a boil, and reduce heat to medium. Cover, and simmer for 20 minutes, stirring occasionally.

Fire Roasted Vegetarian Gumbo

Ingredients

1 serrano pepper
1 banana pepper
1 small jalapeno chile pepper
1/4 cup canola oil
1/4 cup all-purpose flour
2 tablespoons canola oil
2 celery ribs, chopped
1 large onion, chopped
3 green bell peppers, chopped
1 quart vegetable broth
2 cloves garlic, minced
2 tablespoons Cajun seasoning
1 tablespoon smoked paprika
1 tablespoon file powder
1 cup fire-roasted tomatoes
1 sweet potato, peeled and cubed
parsnip, peeled and cubed
1 cup canned red beans, rinsed and drained
1 cup canned black-eye peas, rinsed and drained
2 cups frozen cut okra, thawed

Directions

Preheat oven to broil.

Arrange the serrano, banana, and jalapeno chile peppers on a baking sheet and place in the oven. Watch carefully and broil just until the skins blacken and blister, 4 to 5 minutes. Turn the peppers and continue broiling until all sides are blackened. Remove the peppers from the oven and place in a sealed paper bag to steam. After 15 to 20 minutes, remove peppers from the bag and peel off the crispy black skin. Remove stems and seeds from the peppers, coarsely chop, and place in a bowl.

Heat the canola oil in a large skillet over medium heat until a pinch of flour sprinkled over the oil just begins to bubble. Whisk in the rest of the flour and cook, whisking continuously, until the mixture is well blended and dark brown, about 20 minutes. Once it becomes dark brown, remove the roux from the heat.

Place 2 tablespoons of canola oil into a deep soup pot and heat over medium-high heat. When the oil is just about to smoke, stir in the celery with half of the onions and bell peppers. Cook and stir until the vegetables are tender and the onion is transparent, about 5 minutes. Stir 1/4 cup of the vegetable broth into the pot. Cover, and simmer until almost all the liquid is evaporated, 10 to 15 minutes.

Stir the serrano, banana, and jalapeno chile peppers, along with the uncooked bell peppers and onions, garlic, Cajun seasoning, smoked paprika file powder, into the cooked bell peppers and onions. Stir the roux and 1 cup of stock into the vegetable mixture until the roux dissolves. Cover and simmer 5 minutes. Add the tomatoes, sweet potato, parsnip, red beans, black-eyed peas, okra, and remaining stock. Simmer uncovered 30 minutes more. Season to taste with salt and pepper.

Vegetarian Lentil Spaghetti

Ingredients

1/4 cup dried brown lentils, rinsed and drained
1 (15 ounce) can stewed tomatoes, undrained
1 (15 ounce) can artichoke hearts in water
1/4 teaspoon cayenne pepper, divided
1/4 cup water
3 tablespoons olive oil, divided
1/4 pound thin spaghetti
4 green onions, chopped 1/2 teaspoon sesame seeds salt and pepper to taste

Directions

Place the lentils, tomatoes and artichokes (with the liquid from the cans), 1/8 teaspoon cayenne pepper and the water into a large saucepan. Bring to a boil. Reduce heat to low and simmer until lentils are tender, about 20 minutes.

Meanwhile, bring a large pot of lightly salted water and 1 tablespoon of the olive oil to a boil. Add spaghetti and cook for 8 to 10 minutes or until al dente; drain. Return pasta to pot and cover to keep warm.

Heat remaining 2 tablespoons olive oil in a small skillet over medium heat and cook green onions for about 3 minutes. Add 1/8 teaspoon cayenne pepper and sesame seeds and cook until the seeds are lightly browned, about 2 minutes. Set aside.

Add the lentil mixture to the pot of pasta and toss to distribute evenly. Add the green onion mixture and toss lightly again. Season with salt and pepper to taste.

Vegetarian Shepherd's Pie I

Ingredients

5 russet potatoes, peeled and cut into thirds
4 tablespoons butter
1 1/2 teaspoons salt
ground black pepper to taste
2 cups milk
3 cups water
1/2 cup kasha (toasted buckwheat groats)
2/3 cup bulgur
2 cups chopped onion
2 cloves garlic, minced
2 carrots, diced
2 cups fresh sliced mushrooms
1 1/2 tablespoons all-purpose flour
1 cup whole corn kernels, blanched
3 tablespoons chopped fresh parsley

Directions

Gently boil potatoes in a large pot of water for 20 minutes, or until tender. Drain, and return to the pot. Mash potatoes with 2 tablespoons butter or margarine, 3/4 teaspoon salt, and 1/2 cup milk until fairly smooth. Set aside.

In a saucepan, bring 1 1/2 cups water with 1/2 teaspoon salt to a boil. Stir in kasha. Reduce heat, and simmer, uncovered, for 15 minutes. Add 1 1/2 cups more water, and bring to a boil. Add bulgur, cover, and remove from heat. Let stand for 10 minutes.

In a large saucepan, melt the remaining 2 tablespoons of butter or margarine over medium heat. Add onions, garlic, and carrots; saute until the onions soften. Add mushrooms; cook and stir for 3 to 4 minutes. Sprinkle flour over vegetables; stir constantly for 2 minutes, or until flour starts to brown. Pour remaining 1 1/2 cups milk over the vegetables, and increase heat to high. Stir with a whisk until sauce is smooth. Reduce heat, and simmer for 5 minutes. Stir in corn, 1/4 teaspoon salt, and black pepper to taste.

Mix together vegetable mixture and kasha mixture in a large bowl. Spoon into a buttered 10 inch pie pan, and smooth with a spatula. Spread mashed potatoes over top, leaving an uneven surface.

Bake in a preheated 350 degree F (175 degree C) oven for 30 minutes. Garnish with the chopped parsley, and serve.

Vegetarian Mushroom-Walnut Meatloaf

Ingredients

1 tablespoon olive oil
12 ounces crimini mushrooms, chopped
1 small red onion, finely diced
1 red bell pepper, seeded and diced
1 tablespoon ground sage
1 1/4 cups cooked brown rice
1/2 cup walnuts, finely chopped
1 envelope onion soup mix
1 cup oat bran
1 cup wheat germ
2 egg whites, lightly beaten
1 teaspoon Worcestershire sauce
2 teaspoons prepared mustard

Directions

Preheat oven to 350 degrees F (175 degrees C). Lightly grease a 9x5 inch loaf pan.

Heat the olive oil in a large skillet over medium heat. Stir in the mushrooms, onions, and bell pepper; cook until the onion is transparent, about 5 minutes. Sprinkle sage over the vegetables, and cook until vegetables are soft, about 5 minutes more. Transfer vegetables to a large mixing bowl.

Stir the rice, walnuts, onion soup mix, oat bran, wheat germ, egg whites, Worcestershire sauce, and mustard into the mushroom mixture until thoroughly blended. Spoon into prepared loaf pan, pressing down mixture with a spatula to flatten top.

Bake in preheated oven for 1 hour. Let rest 10 minutes before slicing.

Vegetarian Sandwich Spread

Ingredients

1 (19 ounce) can vegetarian hot dog links
3/4 cup sweet pickle relish
1 onion, chopped
1/2 cup mayonnaise

Directions

In a large bowl mash hot dog links using a potato masher or fork. Blend in relish, onion and mayonnaise.

Vegetarian Cassoulet

Ingredients

2 tablespoons olive oil
1 onion
2 carrots, peeled and diced
1 pound dry navy beans, soaked overnight
4 cups mushroom broth
1 cube vegetable bouillon
1 bay leaf
4 sprigs fresh parsley
1 sprig fresh rosemary
1 sprig fresh lemon thyme, chopped
1 sprig fresh savory
1 large potato, peeled and cubed

Directions

Heat a small amount of oil in a skillet over medium heat. Cook and stir onion and carrots in oil until tender.

In a slow cooker, combine beans, carrots and onion, mushroom broth, bouillon, and bay leaf. Pour in water if necessary to cover ingredients with water. Tie together parsley, rosemary, thyme, and savory, and add to the pot. Cook on Low for 8 hours.

Stir in potato, and continue cooking for 1 hour. Remove herbs before serving.

Vegetarian Lasagna

Ingredients

1 (16 ounce) can diced tomatoes
1 (16 ounce) package instant lasagna noodles
1 bunch fresh spinach, washed and chopped
2 large carrots, shredded
2 large zucchini, diced
2 summer squash, diced
1 large eggplant, diced
1 large head broccoli, cut into florets
2 teaspoons dried oregano
salt and pepper to taste
1 cup shredded mozzarella cheese (optional)
1 cup ricotta cheese (optional)

Directions

Preheat oven to 375 degrees F (190 degrees C). Lightly grease one 9x13 inch baking dish.

Place a layer of tomatoes in the bottom of the baking dish, followed by a layer of noodles, spinach, carrots, zucchini, summer squash, eggplant and broccoli. Season to taste with oregano, salt and pepper. Repeat layering of ingredients until all are used up. If using cheeses sprinkle over broccoli layers and on top of dish.

Bake at 375 degrees F (190 degrees C) for 25 to 35 minutes.

Easy Vegetarian Pasta

Ingredients

1 (16 ounce) package uncooked whole wheat spaghetti
3 tablespoons olive oil
2 tablespoons garlic, minced
3 large tomatoes, diced
1 red onion, chopped
1 yellow bell pepper, chopped
1 red bell pepper, chopped
1 cup chopped zucchini
1/2 cup sliced fresh mushrooms
2 tablespoons balsamic vinegar
2 tablespoons crumbled feta cheese

Directions

Bring a large pot of lightly salted water to a boil. Add pasta and cook for 8 to 10 minutes or until al dente; drain.

Heat the oil in a skillet over medium heat, and saute the garlic until lightly browned. Mix in the tomatoes, onion, yellow bell pepper, red bell pepper, zucchini, and mushrooms. Cook and stir until tender.

Mix the balsamic vinegar into the skillet. Toss with the cooked spaghetti, and sprinkle with feta cheese to serve.

Vegetarian Green Chile Stew

Ingredients

1 tablespoon olive oil
1/4 teaspoon minced garlic
1/2 onion, chopped
2 large carrots, peeled and chopped
1 stalk celery, chopped
4 potatoes, cut in one-inch cubes
1/4 teaspoon chili powder
1/4 teaspoon paprika
1/2 teaspoon salt
1/4 teaspoon pepper
1 yellow squash, cut in one-inch cubes
2 cups packed fresh spinach
1/3 cup frozen corn kernels
1 (16 ounce) can pinto beans, drained
1 cup cooked, shredded spaghetti squash (optional)
2 cups vegetable broth
5 cups water
3 (4 ounce) cans chopped green chile peppers

Directions

Heat olive oil in a large pot over medium-high heat. Add garlic, onion, carrots, celery, potatoes, chili powder, paprika, salt, and pepper. Cook, stirring occasionally, until potatoes are golden brown, about 10 minutes.

Toss yellow squash, spinach leaves, corn, pinto beans, and spaghetti squash into the pot. Continue to stir until spinach leaves have wilted, 1 to 2 minutes.

Pour vegetable broth, water, and green chiles into the mixture. If necessary, add more water to make sure vegetables are covered. Bring stew to a boil, then reduce heat to medium low, cover, and simmer until the vegetables are tender, about 45 minutes.

Vegetarian Gravy

Ingredients

1/2 cup vegetable oil
1/3 cup chopped onion
5 cloves garlic, minced
1/2 cup all-purpose flour
4 teaspoons nutritional yeast
4 tablespoons light soy sauce
2 cups vegetable broth
1/2 teaspoon dried sage
1/2 teaspoon salt
1/4 teaspoon ground black pepper

Directions

Heat oil in a medium saucepan over medium heat. Saute onion and garlic until soft and translucent, about 5 minutes. Stir in flour, nutritional yeast, and soy sauce to form a smooth paste. Gradually whisk in the broth. Season with sage, salt, and pepper. Bring to a boil. Reduce heat, and simmer, stirring constantly, for 8 to 10 minutes, or until thickened.

Delightful Indian Coconut Vegetarian Curry in the

Ingredients

5 russet potatoes, peeled and cut into 1-inch cubes
1/4 cup curry powder
2 tablespoons flour
1 tablespoon chili powder
1/2 teaspoon red pepper flakes
1/2 teaspoon cayenne pepper
1 large green bell pepper, cut into strips
1 large red bell pepper, cut into strips
1 (1 ounce) package dry onion soup mix (such as Lipton®)
1 (14 ounce) can coconut cream
water, as needed
1 1/2 cups matchstick-cut carrots
1 cup green peas (optional)
1/4 cup chopped fresh cilantro

Directions

Place the potatoes into the bottom of a slow cooker.

Mix the curry powder, flour, chili powder, red pepper flakes, and cayenne pepper together in a small bowl; sprinkle over the potatoes. Stir the potatoes to coat evenly. Add the red bell pepper, green bell pepper, onion soup mix, and coconut milk; stir to combine.

Cover the slow cooker and cook on Low until the mixture is bubbling, adding water as needed to keep moist, 3 to 4 hours. Add the carrots to the mixture and cook another 30 minutes. Stir the peas into the mixture and cook until the vegetables are tender to your liking, about 30 minutes. Garnish individual portions with cilantro to serve.

Summer Vegetarian Chili

Ingredients

2 tablespoons extra-virgin olive oil
1 cup chopped red onion
5 large cloves garlic, crushed or minced
2 tablespoons chili powder, or more to taste
2 teaspoons ground cumin
2 cups juicy chopped fresh tomatoes
1 (15 ounce) can no-salt-added black beans, drained
1 cup water (or red wine)
1 cup chopped bell pepper (any color)
1 cup chopped zucchini
1 cup corn kernels
1 cup chopped white or portobello mushrooms
1 cup chopped fresh cilantro, packed
1/8 teaspoon cayenne pepper, or more to taste
Salt and freshly ground black pepper, to taste

Directions

Heat oil in medium pot. Add onion, garlic, chili powder and cumin. Saute over medium heat until onion is soft, about 5 minutes. Add remaining ingredients (except garnishes) and stir. Bring to a boil, then lower heat and simmer 20 minutes or until vegetables are soft. Add more liquid if needed.

Serve alone or over rice (preferably brown). Garnish if desired with any of the following: reduced-fat cheddar cheese, onion, fat-free sour cream, guacamole, fresh cilantro.

Vegetarian Tortilla Dog

Ingredients

1 vegetarian hot dog
1 (6 inch) flour tortilla
1/2 teaspoon margarine
1 slice American cheese

Directions

Place hot dog on a microwave-safe plate and heat on High until warm, about 30 seconds. Place tortilla on a microwave-safe plate, and heat on High until warm, about 15 seconds. Lightly spread the tortilla with margarine. Place the cheese slice on the tortilla, and top with the hot dog. Fold the ends of the tortilla in over the hot dog and roll to close. Heat the tortilla dog in microwave on High until cheese melts, about 30 more seconds.

Malaysian Quinoa (Vegetarian)

Ingredients

1 1/2 cups water, divided
1/2 cup dried soy chunks
(textured vegetable protein)
1 tablespoon peanut butter
1 tablespoon canned cream of
coconut
1/2 bird's eye chile, seeded and
minced
1/2 green onion, diced
1 teaspoon chopped cilantro
1/2 cup uncooked quinoa
salt and pepper to taste

Directions

Boil 1/2 cup water, and pour into a bowl. Mix in soy chunks. Blend in peanut butter, cream of coconut, chile, green onion, and cilantro. Keep warm while the quinoa cooks.

Bring quinoa and remaining 1 cup water to a boil in a pot. Reduce heat to low, cover, and simmer 15 minutes, until quinoa is fluffy. Stir in the soy chunks and peanut butter sauce, and season with salt and pepper to serve.

Vegetarian Chickpea Sandwich Filling

Ingredients

1 (19 ounce) can garbanzo beans, drained and rinsed
1 stalk celery, chopped
1/2 onion, chopped
1 tablespoon mayonnaise
1 tablespoon lemon juice
1 teaspoon dried dill weed
salt and pepper to taste

Directions

Drain and rinse chickpeas. Pour chickpeas into a medium size mixing bowl and mash with a fork. Mix in celery, onion, mayonnaise (to taste), lemon juice, dill, salt and pepper to taste.

Vegetarian Sloppy Joe's

Ingredients

1/4 cup vegetable oil
1/2 cup minced onion
2 (8 ounce) packages tempeh
1/2 cup minced green bell pepper
2 cloves garlic, minced
1/4 cup tomato sauce
1 tablespoon Worcestershire sauce
1 tablespoon honey
1 tablespoon blackstrap molasses
1/4 teaspoon cayenne pepper
1/4 teaspoon celery seed 1/4 teaspoon ground cumin 1/4 teaspoon salt
1/2 teaspoon ground coriander
1/2 teaspoon dried thyme
1/2 teaspoon oregano
1/2 teaspoon paprika
1 pinch ground black pepper
hamburger buns

Directions

Heat oil in a deep, 10-inch skillet over medium-low heat. Cook the onion in the oil until translucent. Crumble the tempeh into the skillet; cook and stir until golden brown. Add the green pepper and garlic; cook another 2 to 3 minutes. Stir in the tomato sauce, Worcestershire sauce, honey, molasses, cayenne pepper, celery seed, cumin, salt, coriander, thyme, oregano, paprika, and black pepper; stir. Simmer another 10 to 15 minutes. Spoon hot onto hamburger buns to serve.

Vibrant Vegetarian Purple Borscht

Ingredients

4 cups water
2 red beets, trimmed and washed
1 1/2 pounds tomatoes, chopped
4 ounces tomato puree
2 tablespoons butter
2 red onions, chopped
2 cups chopped mushrooms
2 carrots, chopped
2 stalks celery, chopped
1/4 cup chopped fresh dill, divided
1 cube vegetable bouillon
2 large yellow potatoes, cubed
1 (15.25 ounce) can kidney beans
6 cups water
1/2 head green cabbage, chopped
1 lemon, juiced
salt and pepper to taste
1 cup sour cream, for topping

Directions

Place the beets into a large pot and cover with 4 cups of water. Bring to a boil over high heat, then reduce heat to medium-low, cover, and simmer until tender, 20 to 40 minutes. Meanwhile, place the tomatoes and tomato puree in a blender and blend until smooth. Set aside.

Meanwhile, heat the butter in a skillet over medium heat. Stir in the onion; cook and stir until the onion has softened and turned translucent, about 5 minutes. Stir in the mushrooms and cook until tender, about 10 minutes. Stir in the carrots, celery, tomato mixture, half of the dill, and the vegetable bouillon. Continue cooking and stirring until the carrots are tender, about 10 minutes.

Remove the beets from the cooking liquid and place them in the freezer in a bowl. Stir the mushroom mixture, potatoes, kidney beans, including the liquid, and 6 cups of water into the beet water. Bring to a boil over high heat, then reduce heat to medium-low, cover, and simmer until the potatoes are tender, about 20 minutes.

Peel, then grate the chilled beets. Stir the beets, cabbage, and remaining dill into the soup. Cover and simmer until the cabbage is tender, about 5 minutes. Stir in lemon juice and season with salt and pepper. Remove from heat and allow soup to rest for at least 2 hours. Bring soup to a boil, and serve hot with a dollop of sour cream.

Vegetarian Turkey Stuffing

Ingredients

1 tablespoon vegetable oil
1 onion, finely chopped
3 stalks celery, finely chopped
1 green bell pepper, finely chopped
1 (4.5 ounce) can mushrooms, drained
1 clove garlic, crushed
salt to taste
ground black pepper to taste
1 1/2 cups corn flake crumbs
1 (10.75 ounce) can condensed cream of mushroom soup

Directions

Preheat oven to 350 degrees F (175 degrees C). Lightly grease a medium casserole dish.

Heat the oil in a skillet over medium heat, and saute the onion, celery, pepper, mushrooms, and garlic until tender. Season with salt and pepper. Mix in the corn flake crumbs and soup. Transfer to the prepared casserole dish.

Bake 30 minutes in the preheated oven, until lightly browned.

Vegetarian Burrito Casserole

Ingredients

3/4 cup white rice
1 1/2 cups water
1 (12 ounce) package frozen soy burger-style crumbles
1 (28 ounce) can whole tomatoes, drained, 1/4 cup juice reserved
2 1/2 teaspoons chili powder
1 teaspoon cumin
1 (1.25 ounce) package taco seasoning mix
2 (10 inch) burrito-size flour tortillas
1 (14.25 ounce) can vegetarian refried beans, divided
2 fresh jalapeno peppers - seeded, sliced, and divided
1 1/2 cups salsa, divided
2 1/2 cups shredded Cheddar cheese, divided

Directions

In a saucepan bring water to a boil. Add rice and stir. Reduce heat, cover, and simmer for 20 minutes.

Preheat oven to 375 degrees F (190 degrees C).

Place soy crumbles, tomatoes, reserved tomato juice, chili powder, cumin, and taco seasoning in a medium frying pan over medium high heat. Cook and stir, breaking up tomatoes, for 10 minutes.

Lay 1 flour tortilla in a lightly greased 8x8 inch baking dish. Layer with one half of the beans, jalapeno slices, rice, salsa, soy mixture, and 1 cup Cheddar cheese. Repeat layers with remaining ingredients, beginning with the flour tortilla, and top with remaining 1 1/2 cups Cheddar cheese.

Bake in the preheated oven for 15 minutes, or until heated through and cheese is melted. Serve immediately.

Grandma's Slow Cooker Vegetarian Chili

Ingredients

1 (19 ounce) can black bean soup
1 (15 ounce) can kidney beans, rinsed and drained
1 (15 ounce) can garbanzo beans, rinsed and drained
1 (16 ounce) can vegetarian baked beans
1 (14.5 ounce) can chopped tomatoes in puree
1 (15 ounce) can whole kernel corn, drained
1 onion, chopped
1 green bell pepper, chopped
2 stalks celery, chopped
2 cloves garlic, chopped
1 tablespoon chili powder, or to taste
1 tablespoon dried parsley
1 tablespoon dried oregano
1 tablespoon dried basil

Directions

In a slow cooker, combine black bean soup, kidney beans, garbanzo beans, baked beans, tomatoes, corn, onion, bell pepper and celery. Season with garlic, chili powder, parsley, oregano and basil. Cook for at least two hours on High.

Vegetarian Nori Rolls

Ingredients

2 cups uncooked short-grain white rice
2 1/4 cups water
1/4 cup soy sauce
2 teaspoons honey
1 teaspoon minced garlic
3 ounces firm tofu, cut into 1/2 inch strips
2 tablespoons rice vinegar
4 sheets nori seaweed sheets
1/2 cucumber, julienned
1/2 avocado, julienned
1 small carrot, julienned

Directions

In a large saucepan cover rice with water and let stand for 30 minutes.

In a shallow dish combine soy sauce, honey and garlic. In this mixture marinate tofu for at least 30 minutes.

Bring water and rice to a boil and then reduce heat; simmer for about 20 minutes, or until thick and sticky. In a large glass bowl combine cooked rice with rice vinegar.

Place a sheet of nori on a bamboo mat. Working with wet hands, spread 1/4 of the rice evenly over the nori; leave about 1/2 inch on the top edge of the nori. Place 2 strips of marinated tofu end to end about 1 inch from the bottom. Place 2 strips of cucumber next to the tofu, then avocado and carrot.

Roll nori tightly from the bottom, using the mat to help make a tight roll. Seal by moistening with water the 1/2 inch at the top. Repeat with remaining ingredients. Slice with a serrated knife into 1 inch thick slices.

Clinton's Special Vegetarian Quiche

Ingredients

1 (17.5 ounce) package frozen puff pastry, thawed
1 cup fresh spinach, cleaned and stemmed
4 tablespoons water
1/4 teaspoon ground nutmeg
1 onion, chopped
2 tablespoons butter
5 eggs
1 cup cottage cheese
1 cup shredded Cheddar cheese
salt and pepper to taste
2 tomatoes, thinly sliced

Directions

Preheat oven to 400 degrees F (200 degrees C). Spray a quiche dish with non-stick cooking spray.

Line the quiche dish with puff pastry, press the pastry firmly in place and trim away any excess pastry. Blind bake for 10 minutes.

In a large skillet place spinach and 4 tablespoons water. Heat the mixture over medium and cover the skillet. Cook until the spinach is done, approximately 2 minutes then drain well. Add nutmeg to the spinach and puree the mixture.

In a large skillet, saute the onion with butter or margarine to taste. Saute until the onions are soft and transparent.

In a medium-size mixing bowl, beat eggs. Stir in the cottage cheese, spinach, and 1/2 cup of cheese. Season with salt and pepper. Arrange onions along the bottom of the pastry-lined quiche dish. Arrange the tomatoes over the onions. Pour the egg-mixture over the onions and tomatoes, and top entire concoction with the remaining cheese.

Bake at 350 degrees F (175 degrees C) for 45 to 50 minutes, or until the quiche has set in the middle. Serve hot or cold, your choice!

Vegetarian Haggis

Ingredients

1 tablespoon vegetable oil
1 medium onion, finely chopped
1 small carrot, finely chopped
5 fresh mushrooms, finely chopped
1 cup vegetable broth
1/3 cup dry red lentils
2 tablespoons canned kidney beans - drained, rinsed, and mashed
3 tablespoons ground peanuts
2 tablespoons ground hazelnuts
1 tablespoon soy sauce
1 tablespoon lemon juice
1 1/2 teaspoons dried thyme
1 teaspoon dried rosemary
1 pinch ground cayenne pepper
1 1/2 teaspoons mixed spice
1 egg, beaten
1 1/3 cups steel cut oats

Directions

Heat the vegetable oil in a saucepan over medium heat, and saute the onion 5 minutes, until tender. Mix in carrot and mushrooms, and continue cooking 5 minutes. Stir in broth, lentils, kidney beans, peanuts, hazelnuts, soy sauce, and lemon juice. Season with thyme, rosemary, cayenne pepper, and mixed spice. Bring to a boil, reduce heat to low, and simmer 10 minutes. Stir in oats, cover, and simmer 20 minutes.

Preheat oven to 375 degrees F (190 degrees C). Lightly grease a 5x9 inch baking pan.

Stir the egg into the saucepan. Transfer the mixture to the prepared baking pan. Bake 30 minutes, until firm.

Vegetarian Stuffed Red Bell Peppers

Ingredients

1 cup quinoa
1 cup water
2 red bell peppers
1/2 Granny Smith apple, cored and chopped
1 tablespoon fresh lime juice
1 teaspoon olive oil
1 clove garlic, minced
1 1/2 tablespoons chopped fresh parsley
1 1/2 tablespoons chopped fresh mint
1 cup chopped tomatoes
3 green onions, thinly sliced
sea salt and pepper to taste

Directions

Bring the quinoa and water to a boil in a saucepan over high heat. Reduce heat to medium-low, cover, and simmer until the quinoa is tender, 20 to 25 minutes.

Preheat oven to 350 degrees F (175 degrees C). Lightly grease a small baking dish. Halve the red peppers lengthwise. Remove the seeds and ribs, but leave the stem intact so the pepper bowls hold their shape; place cut-side-up into the prepared baking dish.

Toss the chopped apple with the lime juice, olive oil, garlic, parsley, mint, tomatoes, and green onions. Fold in the quinoa, and season to taste with salt and pepper. Fill the cut peppers with this mixture, and fill the baking dish with about 1/4 inch of water.

Bake in preheated oven until the peppers are tender, and the quinoa is hot, about 20 minutes.

Vegetarian Kofta Kabobs

Ingredients

1 cup bulgur
2 cups vegetable broth or stock
1 (18.75 ounce) can adzuki beans
2 tablespoons olive oil
1 onion, finely chopped
3 cloves garlic, minced
1 teaspoon ground cumin
1 teaspoon ground coriander
2 tablespoons chopped fresh cilantro
2 teaspoons hot pepper sauce
1 egg, beaten
1 cup stale whole wheat bread cubes
1 cup skim milk
salt and freshly ground black pepper to taste
1 tablespoon olive oil
8 (12-inch) skewers

Directions

Combine the bulgur wheat and vegetable stock in a saucepan. Bring to a boil, then simmer for about 10 minutes, or until liquid has been absorbed. Set aside to cool.

Meanwhile, in a large bowl, combine the adzuki beans, 2 tablespoons of olive oil, onion, garlic, cumin, coriander, cilantro, hot sauce, and the egg. Mash with a potato masher or sturdy whisk until fairly smooth. Soak the bread in milk, then squeeze out the excess; add to the bean mixture along with the bulgur. Mix using your hands until everything is well blended. Cover, and refrigerate for 1 hour, or until firm.

Preheat the oven to 425 degrees F (220 degrees C).

Wet your hands, and form the kofta into 32 oval shapes. Press onto skewers four at a time. Brush with remaining olive oil. Place on a baking sheet or broiling pan.

Bake for 10 to 15 minutes in the preheated oven. Turn over, brush again with oil, and continue baking for 5 to 10 minutes, until crispy.

Vegetarian Split Pea Soup

Ingredients

3/4 cup uncooked orzo pasta
1 cup chopped onion
1 cup chopped celery
2 cloves garlic, minced
1 1/2 cups chopped carrots
1 tablespoon olive oil
1 quart vegetable broth
1 cup dried split peas
1 teaspoon dried thyme
1/2 teaspoon dried chipotle chile pepper
salt and pepper to taste

Directions

Bring a medium-size pot of salted water to a boil, add orzo and cook until al dente. Drain well.

In a large skillet, saute onion, celery, garlic, and carrots in olive oil for 5 minutes.

Place vegetables, vegetable broth, peas, thyme, chile pepper, salt and pepper in a pressure cooker. Cover. When pressure cooker reaches full pressure, cook for 10 to 12 minutes. Remove the pressure cooker from the heat. Add cooked orzo and serve.

Note: If you would like creamier soup, puree soup in a food processor or blender. Add additional broth to bring the soup to the consistency you desire.

Vegetarian Spaghetti

Ingredients

1 (16 ounce) package spaghetti
1 cup chopped onion
1/2 cup chopped celery
1 teaspoon garlic powder
3 tablespoons vegetable oil
1 (26 ounce) jar meatless spaghetti sauce
1 (16 ounce) can garbanzo beans or chickpeas, rinsed and drained
1 (14.5 ounce) can diced tomatoes with garlic and onion, undrained
1 teaspoon sugar
1/2 teaspoon salt
1/2 teaspoon dried oregano
1 bay leaf
1/4 cup grated Parmesan cheese

Directions

Cook spaghetti according to package directions. Meanwhile, in a large skillet, saute the onion, celery and garlic powder in oil until tender. Add the spaghetti sauce, beans, tomatoes, sugar, salt, oregano and bay leaf.

Bring to a boil; cover and simmer for 10 minutes. Discard bay leaf. Drain spaghetti; top with sauce and Parmesan cheese.

Vietnamese Style Vegetarian Curry Soup

Ingredients

2 tablespoons vegetable oil
1 onion, coarsely chopped
2 shallots, thinly sliced
2 cloves garlic, chopped
2 inch piece fresh ginger root, thinly sliced
1 stalk lemon grass, cut into 2 inch pieces
4 tablespoons curry powder
1 green bell pepper, coarsely chopped
2 carrots, peeled and diagonally sliced
8 mushrooms, sliced
1 pound fried tofu, cut into bite-size pieces
4 cups vegetable broth
4 cups water
2 tablespoons vegetarian fish sauce (optional)
2 teaspoons red pepper flakes
1 bay leaf
2 kaffir lime leaves
8 small potatoes, quartered
1 (14 ounce) can coconut milk

2 cups fresh bean sprouts, for garnish
8 sprigs fresh chopped cilantro, for garnish

Directions

Heat oil in a large stock pot over medium heat. Saute onion and shallots until soft and translucent. Stir in garlic, ginger, lemon grass and curry powder. Cook for about 5 minutes, to release the flavors of the curry. Stir in green pepper, carrots, mushrooms and tofu. Pour in vegetable stock and water. Season with fish sauce and red pepper flakes. Bring to a boil, then stir in potatoes and coconut milk. When soup returns to a boil, reduce heat and simmer for 40 to 60 minutes, or until potatoes are tender. Garnish each bowl with a pile of bean sprouts and cilantro.

Vegetarian Kale Soup

Ingredients

2 tablespoons olive oil
1 yellow onion, chopped
2 tablespoons chopped garlic
1 bunch kale, stems removed and leaves chopped
8 cups water
6 cubes vegetable bouillon (such as Knorr)
1 (15 ounce) can diced tomatoes
6 white potatoes, peeled and cubed
2 (15 ounce) cans cannellini beans (drained if desired)
1 tablespoon Italian seasoning
2 tablespoons dried parsley
salt and pepper to taste

Directions

Heat the olive oil in a large soup pot; cook the onion and garlic until soft. Stir in the kale and cook until wilted, about 2 minutes. Stir in the water, vegetable bouillon, tomatoes, potatoes, beans, Italian seasoning, and parsley. Simmer soup on medium heat for 25 minutes, or until potatoes are cooked through. Season with salt and pepper to taste.

Vegetarian Ribs

Ingredients

2 cups gluten
1/3 cup nutritional yeast
2 tablespoons paprika
1 tablespoon salt
2 cups water
1/2 cup smooth peanut butter
1 large onion, minced
1/2 cup olive oil
2 cups barbeque sauce

Directions

In a large bowl, stir together the gluten, yeast, paprika and salt. Pour in the water all at once and quickly mix with a sturdy spoon. Additional water may be necessary to moisten all of the dry gluten. Don't worry that the ball is rather solid, it is supposed to be. Pour off any excess water.

If you want your ribs chewy, leave the ball just as it is. If you want it slightly less chewy, remove it from the bowl and knead for 1 to 2 minutes on a clean surface. Return it to the bowl, and coat with smooth peanut butter. Set aside.

Heat the oil in a skillet over medium heat. Add onion; cook and stir until golden brown. Remove from the heat. Pour the onion and oil over the ball of gluten. Poke a few times with a chopstick, knife or even a fork, allowing the oil to soak into the ball. Let cool.

When the ball is just warm enough to be manageable, use your hands to mix the oil and onions in. There will be a lot of oil that will not mix in and tiny pieces of gluten that will not stay attached. That's okay. The oil mainly helps the gluten absorb the spice. Just mix as much as you can.

Preheat the oven to 350 degrees F (175 degrees C).

Break off good sized handfuls of dough and shape them into strips by pulling and twisting. You want them to be about 4 inches long and 1/2 inch thick. Don't try cutting these, or rolling them out, as that will make them behave more like bread and change the texture appreciably. Place the strips on a greased baking sheet.

Bake for 40 minutes in the preheated oven. Remove from the oven and coat each piece liberally with barbeque sauce. Return to the oven for another 10 minutes.

Vegetarian Stuffed Poblano Peppers

Ingredients

4 poblano peppers
2 tablespoons olive oil
1 (12 ounce) package vegetarian burger crumbles
1 (1.25 ounce) package chili seasoning mix
1/2 cup shredded pepperjack cheese

Directions

Preheat an oven to 350 degrees F (175 degrees C).

Bring a large saucepan of water to a boil. Slice the poblanos in half lengthwise and remove the seeds and stems. Place cleaned peppers in boiling water; cook until soft, about 4 minutes. Drain.

Heat olive oil in a large skillet. Stir in vegetarian crumbles and chili seasoning mix. Cook, stirring, until crumbles are hot, about 5 minutes. Fill the cooked peppers with the seasoned crumbles; top with pepperjack cheese. Arrange stuffed peppers on a baking sheet.

Place peppers in preheated oven until cheese is melted, about 10 minutes.

Al's Quick Vegetarian Spaghetti

Ingredients

1 pound uncooked spaghetti
1 cup broccoli florets
1 (15 ounce) can whole kernel corn, drained
1 cup fresh sliced mushrooms
1 cup sliced carrots
2 (8 ounce) cans tomato sauce

Directions

Bring a large pot of salted water to boil, add spaghetti and return water to a boil. Cook until spaghetti is al dente; drain well.

Combine broccoli, corn, mushrooms, carrots and tomato sauce in large sauce pot. Cook on medium heat for 15 to 20 minutes or until vegetables are tender. Stir occasionally to keep sauce from sticking. Serve sauce over spaghetti.

Vegetarian Chili

Ingredients

2 (15 ounce) cans pinto beans, drained and rinsed
1 (28 ounce) can crushed tomatoes
1 (16 ounce) can kidney beans, rinsed and drained
1 (15 ounce) can yellow hominy, drained
1 (6 ounce) can tomato paste
1 (4 ounce) can chopped green chilies
2 small zucchini, halved and thinly sliced
1 medium onion, chopped
1 1/2 cups water
1 tablespoon chili powder
1 teaspoon ground cumin
1 teaspoon salt
1/2 teaspoon garlic powder
1/2 teaspoon sugar
1/2 cup shredded Monterey Jack cheese

Directions

In a large kettle or Dutch oven, combine the first 15 ingredients; mix well. Bring to a boil. Reduce heat; cover and simmer for 30-35 minutes. Sprinkle with cheese.

Sunday Vegetarian Strata

Ingredients

2 tablespoons olive oil
1/2 pound ground vegetarian breakfast sausage
2 cups chopped onion
2 cloves garlic, minced
1 1/2 cups diced red bell pepper
6 cups cubed whole-wheat country bread
1 tablespoon Dijon mustard
1 1/2 cups grated Swiss cheese
12 large eggs
2 cups 1% milk
1 teaspoon salt, or to taste
freshly ground black pepper to taste

Directions

Heat the olive oil in a large skillet over medium heat and stir in the vegetarian sausage. Cook and stir until the sausage is crumbly, and evenly browned. Stir in the onion, garlic, and bell pepper; cook and stir until softened, 3 to 4 minutes. Remove from heat, and set aside.

Spray a 9x13-inch baking dish with non-stick cooking spray. Arrange bread in an even layer in the prepared baking dish. Scatter the sausage mixture on top. Brush with the Dijon mustard, and sprinkle with cheese. Whisk eggs, milk, salt, and pepper in a large bowl, and pour over the cheese. Cover tightly with plastic wrap, and refrigerate for 2 hours or overnight.

Preheat an oven to 350 degrees F (175 degrees C). Remove strata from the refrigerator, and unwrap.

Bake in the preheated oven until puffed, lightly browned, and the center is set, 1 hour to 1 1/2 hours. Allow to cool for 5 minutes before serving.

Easy Vegetarian Stroganoff

Ingredients

1 (12 ounce) package textured vegetable protein
2 (10.75 ounce) cans condensed cream of mushroom soup
1 (6 ounce) can sliced mushrooms, drained
2 tablespoons minced onion
1 tablespoon garlic powder
1 tablespoon seasoning salt
2 1/2 cups water
1 cup rolled oats
1 tablespoon olive oil

Directions

In a large, heavy skillet over medium heat combine textured vegetable protein, mushroom soup, mushrooms, onion, garlic powder, seasoning salt, water, oats and olive oil. Stir until ingredients are well mixed, oats are moist and soup is dissolved. Reduce heat to low and simmer until thickened, about 10 minutes.

Vegetarian Tourtiere

Ingredients

2 cups vegetable broth
2 cups texturized vegetable protein (TVP)
1/2 cup dried vegetable flakes
3 tablespoons butter
1 cup onion, minced
2 cups mushrooms, minced
2 cups bread crumbs
1 teaspoon freshly cracked peppercorns
1/2 teaspoon sea salt
1/2 teaspoon dried thyme leaves
1/2 teaspoon dried summer savory leaves
1 pinch ground cloves
1 pinch fresh ground nutmeg
1 (12 fluid ounce) bottle beer, room temperature
1 egg, beaten
1 tablespoon milk
2 (9 inch) refrigerated pie crusts
1 teaspoon water

Directions

Pour the vegetable broth into a saucepan and bring to a boil over high heat. Measure the texturized vegetable protein and vegetable flakes into a large mixing bowl. Pour the boiling broth over the texturized vegetable protein and vegetable flakes; soak for 15 minutes.

Meanwhile, melt the butter in a large skillet over medium-high heat, add the mushrooms and onions; cook and stir until soft, about 10 minutes.

Stir the texturized vegetable protein and vegetable flake mixture in with the mushroom and onions. Pour the beer into the skillet with the vegetable mixture; remove from heat and cool.

Preheat oven to 450 degrees F (230 degrees C).

Whisk the egg and milk together in a small bowl.

Line a deep dish pie plate with one round of the prepared pastry. Pour the vegetable mixture into the pastry shell. Prepare the top pastry by cutting a 2 to 3-inch hole in the center of the round using a knife or a decorative cookie cutter.

Moisten the edges of the bottom round with water. Place the top round of prepared pastry on top of the meat filling, pressing around the edges and crimping to seal. Brush the top of the pastry with the egg and milk mixture.

Bake in the preheated 450 degree F (230 degrees C) oven for 15 minutes. Lower the oven temperature to 375 degrees F (190 degrees C) and continue baking until the crust is golden brown, 30 to 40 minutes.

Vegetarian Buffalo Chicken Dip

Ingredients

1 (8 ounce) package seasoned chicken-style vegetarian strips (such as Morningstar Farms® Chik'n Strips), diced
2 (8 ounce) packages reduced fat cream cheese, softened
1 (16 ounce) bottle reduced-fat ranch salad dressing
1 (12 fluid ounce) bottle hot buffalo wing sauce (such as Frank's® REDHOT Buffalo Wing Sauce)
1 cup Colby-Monterey Jack cheese blend

Directions

Place the diced vegetarian chicken strips, cream cheese, ranch dressing, and buffalo wing sauce into a slow cooker. Cook on Low, stirring occasionally, until the cheese has melted and the dip is hot, 1 to 2 hours. Stir in the shredded cheese and serve.

Vegetarian Pasties

Ingredients

3 cups all-purpose flour
1 teaspoon salt
1/2 teaspoon baking powder
1 cup butter
4 eggs
2 teaspoons distilled white vinegar
3 1/2 cups water
1 cup dry lentils
3 potatoes, chopped
1 onion, chopped
1 tablespoon olive oil
1 teaspoon salt

Directions

Preheat oven to 350 degrees F (175 degrees C).

Make the dough: mix flour, salt and baking powder together in a medium size mixing bowl. Cut in butter. Stir in egg, vinegar and 1/2 cup water. Continue stirring until dough is moist enough to be formed into a ball (add more water if necessary). Form the dough into a large ball.

Make the filling: bring a pot of 3 cups water to boil, add lentils and continue to boil for 30 to 45 minutes; until lentils are tender. Watch the lentils and add water if necessary.

Wrap the potatoes in aluminum foil and bake them for 30 minutes in the preheated oven. When the potatoes have cooled cut them into small pieces and mix them with the lentils.

In a frying pan saute onions with oil. Stir the onions into the potato-lentil mixture; season with salt and stir.

Divide the dough into 6 - 8-inch circles. Lay the circles on a flat, floured surface. Place one cup of filling into the center of each circle. Fold the dough around the filling; seal the edges and arrange the pasties on an ungreased cookie sheet. Bake for one hour in the preheated oven.

Vegetarian Link Gravy

Ingredients

6 links vegetarian sausage
3 tablespoons olive oil
1 cup vegetable broth
1/8 cup all-purpose flour
1 teaspoon salt
freshly ground black pepper
1/4 teaspoon dried sage

Directions

Place the vegetarian link or patties and 1 tablespoon oil in a large frying pan, fry the links until done.

Break the links into small pieces. Add the remaining oil and flour to a small pot. Mix the flour with the oil over medium low heat until a rue is formed. Slowly add the vegetable broth, mixing well. Add the salt, pepper, sage and cooked sausage pieces. Bring mixture to a boil.

Vegetarian Chili

Ingredients

1 (12 ounce) package frozen burger-style crumbles
2 (15 ounce) cans black beans, rinsed and drained
2 (15 ounce) cans dark red kidney beans
1 (15 ounce) can light red kidney beans

1 (29 ounce) can diced tomatoes
1 (12 fluid ounce) can tomato juice
5 onions, chopped
3 tablespoons chili powder
1 1/2 tablespoons ground cumin
1 tablespoon garlic powder
2 bay leaves
salt and pepper to taste

Directions

In a large pot, combine meat substitute, black beans, kidney beans, diced tomatoes, tomato juice, onions, chili powder, cumin, garlic powder, bay leaves, salt and pepper. Bring to a simmer and cover. Let the chili simmer for at least 1 hour before serving.

Vegetarian Open Faced Sandwich

Ingredients

6 slices sourdough bread, toasted
3 tablespoons pesto sauce
1 small eggplant, sliced
1 small red bell pepper, sliced
1 medium red onion, sliced
2 tomatoes, sliced
1 cup sliced fresh mushrooms
6 slices mozzarella cheese
4 cloves garlic
dried oregano
dried basil
salt and pepper to taste

Directions

Preheat the oven broiler.

Spread one side of each bread slice with equal amounts pesto sauce. Arrange in a single layer on a baking sheet, pesto side up. Layer each slice with eggplant, red bell pepper, red onion, tomatoes, mushrooms, and cheese. Crush garlic on top of cheese, and season with oregano, basil, salt, and pepper.

Broil 5 minutes in the preheated oven, or until cheese is melted and lightly browned.

Vegetarian Chickpea Curry with Turnips

Ingredients

2 tablespoons olive oil
1/2 onion, diced
2 cloves garlic, minced
1 tablespoon ground cumin
2 tablespoons curry powder
1 (15 ounce) can garbanzo beans (chickpeas), undrained
1/2 red bell pepper, diced
1/2 turnip, peeled and diced
1 cup corn kernels
1/2 (15 ounce) can tomato sauce
1 pinch crushed red pepper flakes (optional)
1 pinch salt
1 pinch cracked black pepper

Directions

Heat the olive oil in a large saucepan over medium heat. Stir in the onion, garlic, cumin, and curry powder; cook and stir until the onion has softened and turned translucent, about 5 minutes. Add the garbanzo beans, red bell pepper, turnip, corn, and tomato sauce. Season with red pepper flakes, salt, and black pepper. Bring to a simmer over medium-high heat, then reduce heat to medium-low, cover, and simmer until the vegetables are tender and the curry has thickened, 1 1/2 to 2 hours.

Vegetarian Southwest One-Pot Dinner

Ingredients

1 1/2 cups dried black-eyed peas, soaked overnight
1 green bell pepper, diced
1 onion, chopped
garlic cloves, chopped
1 (10 ounce) can sweet corn, drained
1 (28 ounce) can diced tomatoes
1/4 cup chili powder
2 teaspoons ground cumin
2 cups cooked rice
1/2 cup shredded Cheddar cheese

Directions

Drain and rinse black-eyed peas thoroughly. Place peas, green pepper, onion, garlic, corn, and tomatoes, in slow cooker. Season with chili powder, and cumin; stir until well blended.

Cover and cook on high for 2 hours. Stir in rice, and cheese. Continue to cook for a further 30 minutes.

Meatiest Vegetarian Chili from your Slow Cooker

Ingredients

1/2 cup olive oil
4 onions, chopped
2 green bell peppers, seeded and chopped
2 red bell peppers, seeded and chopped
4 cloves garlic, minced
1 (14 ounce) package firm tofu, drained and cubed
4 (15.5 ounce) cans black beans, drained
2 (15 ounce) cans crushed tomatoes
2 teaspoons salt
1/2 teaspoon ground black pepper
2 teaspoons ground cumin
6 tablespoons chili powder
2 tablespoons dried oregano
2 tablespoons distilled white vinegar
1 tablespoon liquid hot pepper sauce, such as Tabascoв„ў

Directions

Heat the olive oil in a large skillet over medium-high heat. Add the onions; cook and stir until they start to become soft. Add the green peppers, red peppers, garlic and tofu; cook and stir until vegetables are lightly browned and tender, the whole process should take about 10 minutes.

Pour the black beans into the slow cooker and set to Low. Stir in the vegetables and tomatoes. Season with salt, pepper, cumin, chili powder, oregano, vinegar and hot pepper sauce. Stir gently and cover. Cook on LOW for 6 to 8 hours.

Vegetarian Moussaka

Ingredients

1 eggplant, thinly sliced
1 tablespoon olive oil
1 large zucchini, thinly sliced
2 potatoes, thinly sliced
1 onion, sliced
1 clove garlic, chopped
1 tablespoon white vinegar
1 (14.5 ounce) can whole peeled tomatoes, chopped
1/2 (14.5 ounce) can lentils, drained, juice reserved
1 teaspoon dried oregano
2 tablespoons chopped fresh parsley
salt and pepper to taste
1 cup crumbled feta cheese

1 1/2 tablespoons butter
2 tablespoons all-purpose flour
1 1/4 cups milk
black pepper to taste
1 pinch ground nutmeg
1 egg, beaten
1/4 cup grated Parmesan cheese

Directions

Sprinkle eggplant slices with salt and set aside for 30 minutes. Rinse and pat dry.

Preheat oven to 375 degrees F (190 degrees C).

Heat oil in a large skillet over medium-high heat. Lightly brown eggplant and zucchini slices on both sides; drain. Adding more oil if necessary, brown potato slices; drain.

Saute onion and garlic until lightly browned. Pour in vinegar and reduce. Stir in tomatoes, lentils, 1/2 the juice from lentils, oregano and parsley. Cover, reduce heat to medium-low, and simmer 15 minutes.

In a 9x13 inch casserole dish layer eggplant, zucchini, potatoes, onions and feta. Pour tomato mixture over vegetables; repeat layering, finishing with a layer of eggplant and zucchini.

Cover and bake in preheated oven for 25 minutes.

Meanwhile, in a small saucepan combine butter, flour and milk. Bring to a slow boil, whisking constantly until thick and smooth. Season with pepper and add nutmeg. Remove from heat, cool for 5 minutes, and stir in beaten egg.

Pour sauce over vegetables and sprinkle with Parmesan cheese. Bake, uncovered, for another 25 to 30 minutes.

Vegetarian Phad Thai

Ingredients

1 pound dried rice noodles
2 tablespoons vegetable oil
4 eggs, beaten
2 tablespoons peanut oil
1 1/2 cups peanut butter
1/3 cup water
1/3 cup soy sauce
1 cup milk
1 1/4 cups brown sugar
1/3 cup lemon juice
2 tablespoons garlic powder
1 tablespoon paprika
cayenne pepper to taste
1 pound mung bean sprouts
1 cup shredded carrots
1/4 cup chopped green onions
1/2 cup chopped, unsalted dry-roasted peanuts
1 lime, cut into wedges

Directions

Submerge the rice noodles in a large bowl of hot water for about an hour.

Pour 1/2 tablespoon of oil into a large skillet, and add eggs. Scramble into medium-sized pieces, and transfer to plate. Set aside.

In a saucepan, mix together peanut oil, peanut butter, water, soy sauce, milk, brown sugar, and lemon juice. Season with garlic powder and paprika. Heat until sauce is smooth. Season liberally with cayenne pepper.

Drain noodles; noodles should be very flexible, but still relatively firm. Heat remaining 1 1/2 tablespoons vegetable oil in a large saucepan or wok. Cook noodles in oil, stirring constantly, until they are tender, about 2 minutes.   Stir in peanut sauce, sprouts, carrots, scallions, ground peanuts, and the scrambled eggs. Continue to cook over low heat until vegetables are crisp-tender, about 5 minutes. Serve immediately, garnished with lime wedges.

Vegetarian Pate

Ingredients

1 egg
3 tablespoons vegetable oil
1 large onion, chopped
2 cloves garlic, chopped
20 thin wheat crackers
1/2 cup walnuts
1 (15 ounce) can peas, drained
1/2 teaspoon seasoning salt
salt and pepper to taste

Directions

Place egg in a small saucepan, and cover with cold water. Bring water to a boil, and immediately remove from heat. Cover, and let egg stand in hot water for 10 to 12 minutes. Remove from hot water, cool, peel and chop.

Heat oil in a skillet over low heat, and add chopped onion. Cook, stirring occasionally, until brown and tender. Add chopped garlic, and saute for 1 to 2 minutes. Remove the mixture from the skillet, and set aside to cool.

In a blender or food processor, finely chop wheat crackers and walnuts. Mix in peas, seasoning salt and sauteed onion mixture. Add the egg, and blend to a fine paste, adding water or oil if necessary to attain desired consistency. Season with salt and pepper.

Vegetarian Shepherd's Pie

Ingredients

2 tablespoons extra virgin olive oil, divided
1 large yellow onion, roughly chopped
4 cloves garlic, crushed
2 tablespoons curry powder
2 teaspoons ground cumin
2 small red or green bell peppers, chopped
3 cups cubed eggplant, with peel
1 (15 ounce) can diced tomatoes
1/2 cup water
1 1/4 pounds small red potatoes, halved
1/2 cup fat-free half and half (or milk)
1 cup frozen or fresh peas
1/2 cup grated Parmesan cheese
1 pinch Salt and freshly ground black pepper to taste

Directions

Preheat oven to 400 degrees. In a large skillet over medium heat, heat 1 Tb. oil; add onions, garlic, curry and cumin. Saute until onions are soft, about 5 minutes. Remove to a bowl.

Heat remaining oil in skillet; add peppers, eggplant, tomatoes and 1/2 cup water. Saute until soft, about 20 minutes. Stir in onions. Place in a shallow 8-by-8- inch baking dish.

In a saucepan, boil potatoes until done. Drain and smash. Stir in half and half, peas, salt and pepper. Spread over vegetables and top with Parmesan.

Bake 15 minutes. Brown in broiler. Serve.

Vegetarian Nut Loaf

Ingredients

2 large onions, finely chopped
1 cup chopped fresh mushrooms
1/4 cup finely chopped green pepper
2 tablespoons butter
3 cups grated carrots
1 1/2 cups chopped celery
5 eggs, beaten
1/2 cup chopped walnuts
1/4 cup unsalted sunflower kernels
1/2 teaspoon salt
1/2 teaspoon dried basil 1/2 teaspoon dried oregano 1/4 teaspoon pepper
3 cups soft whole wheat bread crumbs

Directions

In a nonstick skillet, saute onions, mushrooms and green pepper in butter until tender. In a bowl, combine the mushroom mixture, carrots, celery, eggs, walnut, sunflower kernels, salt, basil, oregano and pepper. Stir in bread crumbs:

Coat a 9-in. x 5-in. x 3-in. loaf pan with nonstick cooking spray, then line with waxed paper. Transfer vegetable mixture to a prepared pan. Bake at 350 degrees F for 1 hour or until a meat thermometer reads 160 degrees F Let stand for 10 min before slicing.

Alissa's Vegetarian Lentil Meatloaf

Ingredients

1 1/2 cups French green lentils
3/4 cup chopped onion
1/2 cup shredded carrot
1/2 cup chopped red bell pepper
1/4 cup wheat germ
1/2 cup cooked brown rice
3/4 cup bread crumbs
1/4 cup crushed flax seed
2/3 cup egg whites
1 (6.5 ounce) can tomato sauce
1 tablespoon olive oil
2 teaspoons dried thyme
1 pinch cayenne pepper, or to taste
salt to taste

Directions

Measure the lentils into a saucepan and fill with enough water to cover them by 1 inch. Bring to a boil, and cook until tender, about 45 minutes. Check occasionally and add more water if needed. Drain and set aside to cool.

Preheat the oven to 375 degrees F (190 degrees C). Grease an 8x4 inch loaf pan.

In the bowl of a food processor, combine the onion, carrot, bell pepper and wheat germ. Pulse until finely chopped. Transfer to a bowl. Put the lentils into the food processor and process into a paste. Spoon the lentils into the bowl with the vegetables and mix in the rice, bread crumbs, flax seed, egg whites, tomato sauce and olive oil. Season with thyme, cayenne pepper and salt. Spoon the mixture into the prepared loaf pan.

Bake for 45 minutes in the preheated oven, until heated through and browned on the top. Cool slightly before slicing and serving.

Vegetarian Korma

Ingredients

1 1/2 tablespoons vegetable oil
1 small onion, diced
1 teaspoon minced fresh ginger root
4 cloves garlic, minced
2 potatoes, cubed
4 carrots, cubed
1 fresh jalapeno pepper, seeded and sliced
3 tablespoons ground unsalted cashews
1 (4 ounce) can tomato sauce
2 teaspoons salt
1 1/2 tablespoons curry powder
1 cup frozen green peas
1/2 green bell pepper, chopped
1/2 red bell pepper, chopped
1 cup heavy cream
1 bunch fresh cilantro for garnish

Directions

Heat the oil in a skillet over medium heat. Stir in the onion, and cook until tender. Mix in ginger and garlic, and continue cooking 1 minute. Mix potatoes, carrots, jalapeno, cashews, and tomato sauce. Season with salt and curry powder. Cook and stir 10 minutes, or until potatoes are tender.

Stir peas, green bell pepper, red bell pepper, and cream into the skillet. Reduce heat to low, cover, and simmer 10 minutes. Garnish with cilantro to serve.

Vegetarian White Bean 'Alfredo' with Linguine

Ingredients

1 (16 ounce) package linguine pasta
1/4 cup butter
3 cloves garlic, minced
2 cups cooked navy beans, rinsed and drained
1 1/2 cups soy milk
1 cup asparagus, cut into 1/2-inch pieces
salt and black pepper to taste

Directions

Fill a large pot with lightly salted water, and bring to a boil over high heat. Cook pasta in boiling water, stirring occasionally, until the pasta has cooked through, about 11 minutes. Drain well.

Meanwhile, melt the butter in a large saucepan over medium heat. Stir in the garlic, and cook until golden brown, about 5 minutes. Add 2/3 cup of the beans and 1/2 cup of soy milk; mash with the back of a spoon or a potato masher to create a thick paste. Stir in the remaining soy milk to create a thick sauce. Mix in the remaining beans and asparagus; simmer until asparagus is tender. Season to taste with salt and pepper. Toss pasta with the sauce, and serve.

Vegetarian Cottage Cheese Patties

Ingredients

3 eggs
1 1/2 cups cottage cheese
1 1/2 cups quick rolled oats
3 tablespoons wheat germ (optional)
1 (1 ounce) envelope dry onion soup mix
1 teaspoon dried thyme
2 tablespoons vegetable oil (for frying)
1 (10 ounce) can condensed cream of mushroom soup

Directions

Preheat oven to 350 degrees F (175 degrees C).

Beat eggs into a large bowl. Stir in cottage cheese, rolled oats, wheat germ, dry onion soup mix, and dried thyme. Form into 8 patties.

Heat oil in a skillet over medium heat. Place patties in oil, and brown on both sides. Remove patties to a 9x13-inch baking dish.

Pour condensed soup into a small bowl. Stir in 1/2 can of water (or milk) to dilute, then pour over patties.

Bake in a preheated oven until the soup is bubbly, about 20 minutes.

Convenient Vegetarian Lasagna

Ingredients

2 (12 ounce) packages lasagna noodles
2 pounds ricotta cheese
4 eggs
1 cup grated Parmesan cheese
1/3 cup chopped fresh parsley
2 teaspoons dried basil
ground black pepper to taste
1/2 cup olive oil
1 1/2 cups chopped onion
1 cup sliced carrots
1 1/4 cups chopped green bell pepper
1 (16 ounce) package chopped frozen broccoli, thawed and drained
3 cups chunky-style spaghetti sauce
2 cups shredded mozzarella cheese, divided

Directions

Bring a large pot of lightly salted water to a boil. Add pasta and cook for 8 to 10 minutes or until al dente; drain and set aside.

In a large bowl, combine ricotta cheese, eggs, Parmesan cheese, parsley, basil and ground black pepper. Stir to blend; set aside.

Heat oil in a large saucepan over high heat. Saute onions for about 5 minutes, stirring occasionally; add carrot slices and saute about 2 minutes, then stir in green bell pepper and broccoli. Stir all together, reduce heat to medium and cook until tender, about 5 minutes. Scrape veggies into ricotta mix and mix well.

Preheat oven to 350 degrees F (175 degrees C).

Ladle 1 cup of spaghetti sauce into a 9x13 inch baking dish and spread evenly over the bottom. Place 2 strips of lasagna lengthwise in the dish, then spread about 4 cups of the filling over the pasta. Sprinkle 1 cup of the mozzarella cheese over the filling; repeat layers.

Bake at 350 degrees F (175 degrees C) for 1 hour; let stand about 15 to 20 minutes, to firm up, before serving.

Vegetarian Reubens

Ingredients

1 pound smoked Cheddar cheese, shredded
1 cup thousand island salad dressing, or to taste
1 (16 ounce) jar sauerkraut, drained
12 slices dark rye bread
2 tablespoons butter
2 tomatoes, sliced

Directions

In a large mixing bowl, stir together the cheese and sauerkraut. Add enough dressing to coat, and mix thoroughly.

Butter each slice of bread on one side. Spread a thick layer of the cheese mixture onto unbuttered side of half of the bread slices. Top with sliced tomato and another slice of bread.

Heat a large skillet to medium-high heat. Fry sandwiches on both sides until the outside is toasted and the cheese is melted.

Farmer's Market Vegetarian Quesadillas

Ingredients

1/2 cup chopped red bell pepper
1/2 cup chopped zucchini
1/2 cup chopped yellow squash
1/2 cup chopped red onion
1/2 cup chopped mushrooms
1 tablespoon olive oil
cooking spray
6 (9 inch) whole wheat tortillas
1 1/4 cups shredded reduced-fat sharp Cheddar cheese

Directions

In a large nonstick pan, cook red pepper, zucchini, yellow squash, onion, and mushrooms in olive oil over medium to medium-high heat for about 7 minutes, or until just tender. Remove vegetables from pan.

Coat the same pan with cooking spray, and place one tortilla in pan. Sprinkle 1/4 cup of cheese evenly over tortilla, and layer 3/4 cup of the vegetable mixture over the cheese. Sprinkle another 1/8 cup of cheese on the vegetables, and top with a second tortilla. Cook until golden on both sides, for approximately 2 to 3 minutes per side. Remove quesadilla from pan, and repeat with remaining ingredients. Cut each quesadilla into 8 triangles with a pizza cutter. Serve hot.

Vegetarian Stuffing

Ingredients

1 (1 pound) loaf day-old bread, torn into small pieces
1 (10.75 ounce) can condensed cream of mushroom soup
1 (10.5 ounce) can vegetable broth
2 tablespoons water
1 teaspoon poultry seasoning
salt to taste
ground black pepper to taste
1/2 cup wild rice, cooked (optional)
1/4 cup dried cranberries (optional)
1/2 cup fresh mushrooms (optional)
1/2 cup chopped pecans (optional)
1/4 cup cubed apples (optional)

Directions

Mix together the bread, cream of mushroom soup, vegetable broth, water, poultry seasoning, and salt and pepper to taste. Add any or all of the optional ingredients as desired. It will be sticky. Shape into a loaf and wrap in (nonstick, sprayed) foil to bake.

Bake for about an hour at 350 degrees F (175 degrees C). You can slice it like a meatloaf and serve.

The Best Vegetarian Chili in the World

Ingredients

1 tablespoon olive oil
1/2 medium onion, chopped
2 bay leaves
1 teaspoon ground cumin
2 tablespoons dried oregano
1 tablespoon salt
2 stalks celery, chopped
2 green bell peppers, chopped
2 jalapeno peppers, chopped
3 cloves garlic, chopped
2 (4 ounce) cans chopped green chile peppers, drained
2 (12 ounce) packages vegetarian burger crumbles
3 (28 ounce) cans whole peeled tomatoes, crushed
1/4 cup chili powder
1 tablespoon ground black pepper
1 (15 ounce) can kidney beans, drained
1 (15 ounce) can garbanzo beans, drained
1 (15 ounce) can black beans
1 (15 ounce) can whole kernel corn

Directions

Heat the olive oil in a large pot over medium heat. Stir in the onion, and season with bay leaves, cumin, oregano, and salt. Cook and stir until onion is tender, then mix in the celery, green bell peppers, jalapeno peppers, garlic, and green chile peppers. When vegetables are heated through, mix in the vegetarian burger crumbles. Reduce heat to low, cover pot, and simmer 5 minutes.

Mix the tomatoes into the pot. Season chili with chili powder and pepper. Stir in the kidney beans, garbanzo beans, and black beans. Bring to a boil, reduce heat to low, and simmer 45 minutes. Stir in the corn, and continue cooking 5 minutes before serving.

Lightning Source UK Ltd.
Milton Keynes UK
UKHW052217150221
378843UK00008B/1042